MODERN MONOGRAPHS IN INDUSTRIAL MEDICINE   6

Editor in Chief: ANTHONY J. LANZA, M.D.
Consulting Editor: RICHARD H. ORR, M.D.

A Manual of Neurology and Psychiatry in Occupational Medicine

By RALPH T. COLLINS, A.B., M.D., Med.Sc.D.

Consultant, Neurology and Psychiatry,
Eastman Kodak Company, Rochester, New York

GRUNE & STRATTON   •   1961

NEW YORK AND LONDON

OTHER BOOKS IN THE MODERN MONOGRAPHS IN INDUSTRIAL MEDICINE SERIES

1. Noise and Your Ear. *Aram Glorig*
2. Alcoholism. *Arnold Z. Pfeffer*
3. Rehabilitation in Industry. *Donald A. Covalt*
4. Industrial Carcinogens. *Robert E. Eckardt*
5. Radiation. Use and Control in Industrial Application. *Charles W. Shilling*

Contents

Foreword

THIS BOOK can best be designated as a handbook or guide for occupational physicians to aid them in recognizing and dealing with neuropsychiatric diagnoses. To us it seems altogether encouraging that such a useful manual is being published. It should have wide usefulness not only for those physicians in occupational medicine, but for the general practitioner as well, and particularly in relation to the increasing role he is playing in providing occupational health service to people who work with smaller employment groups.

The author points out in the introductory chapter that it is not intended as a text book but rather a manual of practical considerations for helping the occupational physician orient and aid himself in deciding whether he is confronted with a neurological or psychiatric problem and what to do about it. The outlines for a quick rundown of symptoms and findings and diagnoses should prove most helpful.

During the years we have been engaged in an effort to place and adjust employees of differing personalities and capacities in a wide variety of environments, we have frequently wished for such help as this book can give.

Dr. Collins begins the chapters on psychiatry with the statements we are all familiar with but which is impressive no matter how many times it is repeated: "Emotional illnesses cause more absenteeism than all other illnesses save the common cold." If the occupational physician can help the worker to attain emotional stability, he will be doing a great deal for all concerned. An emotionally well balanced work group should mean much in the success of any organization.

We agree that out and out mental cases should be dealt with by psychiatrists, but as for the larger group of personality disorders, who are such prolific sources of "health problems," "attendance problems," "production problems," and "disciplinary problems," the occupational physician with proper psychiatric orientation, as outlined here, can many times do very well.

Years ago, Dr. V. V. Anderson, pioneer occupational psychiatrist for R. H. Macy Company, concluded that the occupational physician is being depended upon more and more for aid in dealing with matters other than just the treatment of the sick and injured. "Issues affecting the personnel value of employees; matters relating to the effects of certain jobs in producing fatigue or influencing the health of workers; medical matters affecting employment, placement, training and management — will more and more in the future be referred to him. He needs a technique that will enable him to review scientifically the whole case, the entire individual, and not just a part of him. A training in psychiatry is a fundamental need of industrial physicians."

This opportunity for such "know how" Dr. Collins has ably outlined.

We know of no one better able, nor better qualified than Dr. Collins to select the material for a manual relating neuropsychiatric conditions to occupation. He has had a broad and diversified background, tempered with many years of first-hand experience in an active in-plant health program, with an exceptional interest and participation in voluntary health agency activities in the community, and with an outstanding leadership role in stimulating and developing the needed bond between neurology-psychiatry and the problems of people who work.

William A. Sawyer, M.D.
Former Medical Director
Eastman Kodak Company

James H. Sterner, M.D.
Medical Director
Eastman Kodak Company

Preface and Acknowledgment

THIS MANUAL is intended to aid physicians at the work place in industry or in any other occupational setting with some of the neurologic and psychiatric problems which may occur in their practice. Since this is not a textbook, I have been limited in space. However, this limitation has forced me to be brief and practical which I believe is what a busy occupational physician would wish. Therefore, there is much material in outline form, in columns, in questions and in tables. In condensing material and in choice of material in a short book, an author cannot please everyone. Undoubtedly, I have left out topics which should be included, but perhaps these can be added in subsequent editions. I have tried to present the subject in language which is readily understood.

The author acknowledges with thanks the following authors, publishers and other copyright owners who have given permission for direct quotations and/or for rearrangement of published material.

1. Bond, Dougles D., Flumerfelt, J. M., and Bidder: Quotes on interviewing, section on psychiatry. The Specialties in General Practice, ed. 2, edited by Cecil, R. L. and Conn, H. F. Courtesy of W. B. Saunders Co., 1957, p. 174, Philadelphia.

2. Brock, S.: Adaptation of material from Injuries of the Brain and Spinal Cord, ed. 4. Courtesty of The Springer Publishing Company, Inc., New York.

3. Collins, Ralph T.: Quotation on pages 210-212 from "Are You Accident Prone?" Courtesty of This Week Magazine, United Newspapers Magazine Corporation, publishers, December 11, 1960, New York.

4. Collins, Ralph T.: Quotation on page 223 from We Hire the Whole Man. Courtesty of the Rotarian Magazine publishers, May 1956.

5. Collins, Ralph T.: Quotation on pages 66-71 and 185-189 from article Optimum Time Off From Work for Neurologic and Psychiatric Disabilities. Courtesty of Industrial Medicine and Surgery, Vol. 25, September 1956, No. 9, pages 408-412.

6. Engel, George L.: Section on Fainting, pages 51-53 from monograph on Fainting — Physiological and Psychological Considerations, ed. 2, 1961. Courtesy of Charles C Thomas, Springfield, Ill.

7. Fetterman, J.: Quotation on pages 198, 199 and adaptation of material from The Mind of the Injured Man. Courtesty of Industrial Medicine Book Company, 1943, Chicago.
8. Golin, Milton: quotes on p. 204 from The Troubled Employee. The Journal of the American Medical Association, November 8, 1959.
9. Grinker, Roy: Quotation on p. 47 and adaptation of material from Neurology, ed. 5. Courtesy of Charles C Thomas, Springfield, Ill.
10. Haymaker, Webb and Woodhall, B.: Quotations and use of illustrations and charts on pages 110-131 from Peripheral Nerve Injuries, ed. 1. Courtesy of W. B. Saunders Company, 1945, Philadelphia.
11. Kent, G. H.: Quotation on page 157-158 from Oral Test for Emergency Use in Clinics, Mental Measurement Monographs No. 9. Courtesy of Williams & Wilkins, 1932, Baltimore.
12. Ling, T. M.: Quotation on pp. 134, 135 from Mental Health and Human Relations in Industry. Courtesy of H. K. Lewis & Co. Ltd., 1954, London.
13. McLean, Alan, and Taylor, Graham.: Quotations on pages 224-226 by permission from Mental Health in Industry. Courtesy of McGraw Hill Book Company, Inc., Blakiston Division, 1958, New York.
14. McKendree, C. A.: Adaptation of material from Neurological Examination. Courtesy of W. B. Saunders Company, 1928, New York.
15. Pfeffer, Arnold Z.: Quotations and adaptations of material on pages 212-216, from Alcoholism, Modern Monographs in Industrial Medicine. Courtesy of Grune and Stratton, publishers, 1958, New York.
16. Ross, W. Donald: Quotations and adaptation of material on pages 208-210 from Practical Psychiatry for Industrial Physicians. Courtesy of Charles C Thomas, 1956, Springfield, Ill.
17. Sadler, William S.: Adaptation of material on pages 159-172 from Modern Psychiatry. Courtesy of C. V. Mosby Company, 1945, St. Louis.
18. Taylor, Graham: Quotations on pages 77-81 from report No. 36. Courtesy of Taylor, Graham, Chairman, Committee on Psychiatry

in Industry, Group for the Advancement of Psychiatry, 1957, New York.

19. Wechsler, I. S.: Quotations on pages 46, 47, 200, 201 from Textbook of Clinical Neurology, ed. 7. Courtesy of W. B. Saunders Company, 1952, New York.

20. World Health Organization: Quotations and adaptation of material on pages 160, 161 from Manual of the International Statistical Classification of Disease, Injuries and Causes of Death, Seventh Revision of the International Lists of Diseases and Causes of Death, World Health Organization, Geneva, Switzerland, 1955.

Much encouragement and advice were given me by Dr. Anthony J. Lanza, Emeritus Professor and Head, Department of Industrial Medicine, New York Post Graduate Medical School, throughout the preparation of this manual. The author is indeed grateful for such counsel. In the early stages, Dr. Richard H. Orr, former consulting editor, Modern Monographs in Industrial Medicine, contributed to the over-all style of the manual and the author appreciates his suggestions. Substantial parts of the manuscript were read by Dr. S. Bernard Wortis, Professor of Neurology and Psychiatry and Dean, College of Medicine, New York University, and the author is grateful to him. Dr. James H. Sterner and Dr. William A. Sawyer offered many helpful suggestions and both read the complete manuscript. Dr. Charles Lewis and Dr. David W. Fassett deserve my thanks for their contribution to the preparation of the material on chemical agents and their effect on the nervous system.

A special thank you is due to the secretaries who have faithfully and devotedly given of their services to the preparation of this manual, viz: Miss Shirley Smith, Miss Marilyn Love and Mrs. Marjorie Bailey.

Ralph T. Collins, M.D.

To my father
Charles E. Collins, M.D.
and my mother
who inspired me years ago

and to my wife, Neva
and Ralph Jr., Camille Ann and Pamela Jo
who inspire me today

1.   *Neurology at the Work Place (Occupational Neurology)*

NEUROLOGIC PROBLEMS are bound to appear sooner or later in any occupational practice. However, they will not be as numerous as psychiatric problems and their detection will depend on the interest, the alertness and the diagnostic acumen of the occupational physician. To a neurologist certain symptoms and signs have meaning in the light of his experience as far as localization and pathology are concerned. To the interested occupational physician, certain signs and symptoms may not have the same meaning, but they could have a general meaning pointing the way to further neurologic investigation. The following chapters on neurology in the work place are not intended to be a textbook of neurology. It is hoped that they may present a few practical points to help the occupational physician orient and aid himself to decide whether he has a neurologic problem and what to do about it.

In my experience, the following neurologic conditions appear in the occupational setting with enough regularity to warrant knowledge enough for recognition, viz: multiple sclerosis; epilepsy; peripheral neuritides, such as radial, ulnar, sciatic, femoral, cutaneous, brachial and peroneal; migraine; atypical facial neuralgia; Bell's palsy; optic neuritis; retrobulbar neuritis; diplopia due to a virus infection; acute labrynthitis; Meniere's syndrone; cerebrovascular disease manifested by gross disturbance of motor and sensory function or by more localized areas of disturbance; hypertensive brain disease (encephalopathy); spontaneous hypoglycemia; brain tumors; paralysis agitans; and rupture of intervertebral discs. The following neurologic conditions have been seen with less frequency, viz: Amyotrophic lateral sclerosis, progressive muscular atrophy, subacute combined degeneration of the spinal cord, progressive muscular dystrophy, myotonia acquisita, scalenus anticus syndrome, carotid sinus syndrome, spasmodic torticolis and meralgia paresthetica.

When a neurologic condition is discovered at the pre-employment examination or during the course of employment, the occupational physician must decide whether the individual will be able to do the job for which he was hired and whether he will be able to continue his present employment at the same or another job. If the occupational physician needs some help in the handling of the neurologic case from a diagnostic, therapeutic or placement viewpoint, he may refer the employee to a neurologist in the community, if his company does not have a neurologist on the medical staff. If the employee develops a progressive degenerative type of neurologic condition, the occupational physician must then decide whether he can continue to work at his same job, or whether another job will be suitable for his reduced working efficiency. He, the occupational physician, may consult with the employee's supervisor and with the personnel department to appraise them as to the medical fitness of the employee to continue on a specific job. As the disease progresses, it may be necessary to have the individual move to an easier and less exacting job. Most companies will feel a moral responsibility and a deep concern for such an individual and will try in every way to make his job as comfortable as possible. There should be no job transfer unless the medical department is notified first. When an employee develops an acute neurologic condition such as sciatic neuritis, brachial neuritis or a rupture of an intervertebral disc, he may be assigned to a less exacting job when he returns from his acute illness or from his operation. Constant and repeated examinations will be carried on by the occupational physician to gauge his ability to engage in a graduated increase in his work load and responsibility.

The occupational physician working in companies which manufacture or deal in such various chemical compounds as the organo-metallic compounds, should be aware of the effects of these various chemicals on the central nervous system. These will be discussed in Chapter 8.

There may be some occupational physicians who will profess lack of knowledge and some frustration in the face of a suspected neurologic disease process. They will be reminded of their medical school days when neurology was taught sparingly. However, there will be occupational physicians who will have to develop insights and knowledge in neurology and, as we shall see later, into psychiatry also, because they will be operating in a community far afield from the metropolitan areas where neurologists and psychiatrists are located. The occupational physician will find it very rewarding personally when he becomes sufficiently adept to make a neurologic diagnosis and to follow through in treatment and in the handling of the patient. It is suggested for those who are interested in learning more about neurology and neurologic conditions to consult the following textbooks:

REFERENCES

1. Wechsler, I. S.: A Textbook of Clinical Neurology, ed. 7. Philadelphia, W. B. Saunders Co., 1952.
2. Grinker, R. R., Bucy, P. C., and Sahs, A. L.: Neurology, ed. 5. Springfield, Ill., Charles C Thomas, 1960.
3. Merritt, H. H.: A Textbook on Clinical Neurology, ed. 2. Philadelphia, Lea & Febiger, 1959.
4. Brock, S.: The Basis of Clinical Neurology. Baltimore, William Wood & Co., 1937.
5. Haymaker, W., and Woodhall, B.: Peripheral Nerve Injuries, Philadelphia, W. B. Saunders Co., 1945.
6. McKendree, C.A.: Neurological Examination. Philadelphia, W. B. Saunders Co., 1928.
7. Nielsen, J. M.: A Textbook of Clinical Neurology, ed. 3. New York, Paul B. Hoeber, 1951.

2. *Neurologic History Reminders*

WHEN THE OCCUPATIONAL PHYSICIAN senses that he may have a neurologic problem, he should then begin taking a systematic neurologic history. Each physician will have developed a method of his own to cover the salient neurologic facts needed for a diagnosis as a result of his medical school teaching in neurology and his subsequent clinical experience. However, there may be few physicians who may not have had sufficient neurologic teaching in medical school or who may have become a little rusty in this regard. The following method of taking a neurologic history is one that has proven adequate for the author. Whatever the method, each physician should have a method and stick to it from day to day. If one aspect is left out, soon others will be left out and the history will lack sufficient information to make a definitive diagnosis. Consistency in history and in neurologic examination is difficult to maintain, but it will pay off in the end. One is tempted at times to take short cuts because of lack of time. This should be avoided. The patient should be asked to return for another visit so that more time can be spent in a methodical taking of the history. If time is short at the first meeting with the patient, the neurologic examination might be postponed until the next visit, if the situation is not urgent.

The patient should be asked to tell his story in his own way without any interruptions. Questions about what he says and what he does not say should be left until he has finished. Sometimes, important clues are lost if premature questioning occurs. Watch the patient closely as he tells his story for signs of restlessness, emotional upset, depression, anxiety, irritability, and other signs of disorders of thinking, feeling and behavior. After the patient has told his story, direct questioning may begin about various symptoms and organ systems. *At the end of this chapter is a list of pertinent neurologic questions which have proved valid in any general neurologic condition.* The following general questions might be considered, viz.:

1. How long have you noticed this complaint?
2. Has it been constant or does it come and go?
3. Has anyone in your family had anything like this?
4. Have you had any injuries? Any accidents?

5. Have you had any infections of late?
6. Have you ever had this complaint before?
7. Did you have the complaint come on suddenly or gradually?

It is natural, of course, to center the questioning around the part of the body involved in the complaint, such as the head, the eyes, the ears, the neck, the shoulders, the arms, legs, etc. The symptoms may also center around functions of the body such as vision, hearing, talking, smelling, tasting, thinking, writing, the use of the hands and of the legs, and of walking and maintaining balance.

The author was taught in his neurologic training to take a history by topography of the body rather than by neurologic systems. Therefore, we shall start with the head and finish with the feet. As one receives answers to these questions, one should begin to think of neurologic diagnostic possibilities. The neurologic conditions mentioned in this chapter are the most likely ones to think about. As one's experience grows, one will be able to point one's thinking to a few important probabilities. In this book I shall mention only the *common* neurologic conditions and I refer the reader to textbooks of clinical neurology for a more comprehensive treatment of complete differential diagnosis.

If one cannot make a diagnosis after taking a history and doing a neurologic examination, one might start in again and take another complete neurologic history. This method may commonly lead to a diagnosis. One often uses different approaches to the problem of the main complaint, and, as association of ideas develop in the minds of the patient and physician, this may lead into different areas of thinking and to placing the emphasis on this or that point differently.

The following neurologic symptoms should be considered in taking a neurologic history. I have suggested a few questions to ask about each symptom and a few conditions which might be considered in one's thinking of differential diagnoses.

HEADACHE

Questions

Continuous, intermittent, location, type, relation to posture, sudden or slow onset, associated with nausea and/or vomiting, following an injury, associated with or preceded by visual scotomata, following an emotional situation?

Interpretation

1. *Head injury* — tends to be located at the site of the injury, is aggravated by the upright position, relieved by lying down, may last many weeks or months, but generally diminishes in intensity and frequency.

2. *Vascular insult* — sudden onset is the rule, motor and/or sensory signs usually occur on one side of the body in a cerebral hemorrhage or thrombosis, such as, weakness of one side of the face and arm or a segment of an arm or leg together with possibly a "numb" or "prickly" feeling on one side of the body. There may be a history of hypertension.

3. *Migraine* — usually is one sided and occurs following visual symptoms as scintillating scotomata, family history usually is present, nausea and/or vomiting may occur, entire syndrome usually follows an emotional stress or strain, the personality of a patient with migraine includes the following factors which have been described as: driving, conscientious, sensitive and serious minded.

4. *Tension* — headaches which build up during the day from tension, stress, strain, and worry usually are located in one region of the head — base of the skull, upper neck, one temple area, etc.

5. *Brain tumor* — headaches becoming progressively worse with time, not relieved well with ordinary analgesics or change of posture, occurring during the night or early morning hours, accompanied usually with nausea and/or vomiting and slow pulse. Neurologic signs and symptoms from preasure and irritation may also be present.

6. *Subdural hematoma* — localized headache following a head injury, some weeks or months before. Neurologic symptoms and signs may also be present.

7. *Postural headaches* — postural hypotension may be present.

BUMPS ON THE HEAD

Questions

Have you noticed any bumps or lumps on your head lately? If so, when did the lump occur? Is it tender? Does it get smaller or larger? Has it grown larger since you first noticed it?

Interpretation

1. *Injury* — following an injury a hematoma may have been present which would recede in time.

2. *Brain tumor* — a brain tumor lying on the surface of the brain may erode the inner table of the skull and gradually push the overlying bone tissue up causing a bump on the skull.

3. *Wen* — patients who have multiple wens throughout the body may have one or more on the scalp. These are benign of course.

TENDER AREAS OF THE HEAD

Questions

When did you first notice tenderness? Has it been getting worse? Had any injury lately? Does it hurt when you comb your hair?

Interpretation

1. *Skull injury* — recent injury or a few weeks previously suggesting a growing subdural hemotoma.
2. *Brain tumor* — erosion of the skull by a brain tumor as a meningioma.

HISTORY OF UNCONSCIOUSNESS IN THE PAST

Questions

How did it happen? How long were you unconscious? Do you remember what happened just before and just after you became unconscious? Were you in the hospital and how long? Did you have a spinal puncture? Were x-rays taken in the hospital? What were the reports of all of these procedures? Did you have a head injury? Any bleeding from the nose, ears or mouth?

Interpretation

1. *Brain injury* — the greater the injury the deeper the unconsciousness. Bleeding from the nose, ears, or mouth may have also occurred and usually signifies fractures at the base of the skull.
2. *Convulsive disorder* — may be caused from diverse causes. See below.
3. *Carotid sinus syndrome* — usually occurs on a twisting or bending of the neck in various positions with a tight collar around the neck.
4. *Hypotensive states* — low blood pressure and sudden changes in posture may cause these.
5. *Emotional conditions* — patients usually not truly unconscious and there are elements of hysteria present and a history of emotional instability.
6. *Nutritional deficiencies.*
7. *Cerebral hemorrhage or thrombosis*
8. *Brain tumor*

CONVULSIVE DISORDERS

Questions

Ever had fits before; fainting spells, weak spells, convulsions, unconscious spells, turning spells, etc.? Ever had any convulsions on one side of the body? It is well to remember that people call a convulsion by many different names and often by a colloquial local expression. People will often deny having any spells unless one asks them specifically if they have had what the person has called them. Since one is not a mind reader, one should ask the question of convulsions in many different ways until one is sure that the patient understands. If the patient is an applicant, the applicant may deny convulsions in order to obtain a job. There are still many employers who will deny jobs to people with a convulsive disorder. Convulsions which begin for the first time after the age of 20 years should be considered symptomatic of some organic disease of the brain unless proven otherwise. Brain tumor or cerebral atrophy are two of the most common causes of convulsions in later life.

Interpretation

1. *Brain tumors* — a generalized convulsion is commonly a first symptom. However, a brain tumor may cause a contralateral one sided convulsion involving a side of the face or an arm or a leg. This type of convulsion is called a Jacksonian convulsion, named from the neurologist who first described it.

2. *Hypoglycemia* — generalized convulsions occurring early in the morning from about 4 a.m. are suspect of spontaneous hypoglycemia. Blood sugar estimation should be taken.

3. *Head injury* — scar tissue in the cerebral cortex at the site of a previous head injury will occasionally produce generalized or localized convulsions. An electroencephalogram might help to localize the scarred or epileptogenous area.

4. *Subdural hematoma* — the gradual development of a post traumatic subdural hematoma often will produce a generalized or localized convulsion. This emphasizes the importance of ascertaining if there has ever been a head injury in the presence of convulsions.

5. *Cerebral atrophy* — gradual development of symptoms of cerebral deterioration such as, memory impairment, poor judgement, personality changes, irritability, confusion, and disorientation. Convulsions may be first symptom. Occurs from 50 years of age.

6. *Psychogenic* — the character of a "convulsion" differs from the typical and usually has a bizarre, cautious note about it. The setting is usually one of stress or strain, the fall is often a "planned" one in which injuries are avoided, no bruises resulting, no biting of the tongue or urinary incontinence, and no drowsiness following the "fit."

DIZZINESS

Questions

Ever been light headed or dizzy? When? Where? How often? In what body position? Has the room ever gone around you or have you ever gone around the room? Where you nauseated or did you vomit during your dizzy spell? Had you had an upper respiratory infection at that time such as a head cold or a sore throat or a sinus infection or an earache? Any other illnesses at the time of your attacks of dizziness? Did you have poor hearing at the time of your dizziness? (Meniere's)

Interpretation

1. *Vertigo* — accompanies inner ear pathology and produces body disorientation with gastric symptoms.

2. *Head injuries* — dizziness occurs often following head injuries as part of the post-traumatic head syndrome.

3. *Psychogenic* — emotional disorders are usually present.

VISUAL DISTURBANCES

Questions

Has your vision been reduced lately? Any double vision? Have you seen one-half of a newspaper page while reading or bumped into door jambs on one side as you go through the doorway? Any blind spots in your vision? When did you have your eyes examined last? How often do you have your eyes examined? Have you had any stronger glasses prescribed for you during the past few years?

Interpretation

1. *Errors of refraction* — a refraction would restore vision.

2. *Brain tumor* — increased intracranial pressure will reduce vision generally and later in the course of the brain tumor might cause weakness of the ocular nerves, mainly the abducens or the sixth cranial nerve which will then cause diplopia. Pressure from a brain tumor on visual pathways will produce visual field defects which can usually be plotted out such as hemianopsia, quadrantanopsia.

3. *Multiple sclerosis* — patient will usually complain of blurred vision, double vision or areas of blindness in one or both eyes. These visual disturbances may come and go over a period of weeks or months. Patient is usually between the ages of 20 and 40 years of age and has other symptoms and signs such as cerebellar or pyramidal tract disturbances.

4. *Hysteria* — may have double vision in *one* eye or may have many bizarre visual complaints of fogging, fading, a veil over the eyes, etc., and will have a personality disturbance consonant with hysteria.

5. *Amblyopia ex anopsia* — may have had poor vision since birth or early development in one eye because of strabismus so that only one eye was used for vision in order to blot out double vision. The optic nerve of the unused eye atrophies from disuse.

6. *Retrobulbar neuritis* — unilateral or bilateral, pain in or behind the eye, difficulty in vision (the patient sees nothing and the doctor sees nothing is an old saying about this condition), later optic atrophy is found — usually caused by some infection (virus) or intoxication, such as tobacco or alcohol.

7. *Optic neuritis* — blurred vision, pain in the eye and reduced vision. The optic disc will usually be inflamed and the margins will be obscured.

HEARING DISTURBANCES

Questions

Any trouble hearing lately? Any ringing in the ears? Abscesses in the ears? Punctured ear drums? Wax in the ears? Ever had the ears lanced? Any pain in the ears or behind the ears? Any infections of the nose or throat or sinuses lately?

Interpretation

1. *Otosclerosis* — gradual reduction in hearing beginning at an early age in one or both ears, usually accompanied by tinnitus and vertigo.

2. *Eighth nerve tumor* — gradual reduction in hearing in one ear with subsequent symptoms of involvement of nerve tissue in the vicinity of the eighth nerve, such as facial weakness on the same side of the hearing loss. Later, as intracranial pressure increases, symptoms of headache, nausea, vomiting, double vision and contralateral motor and sensory symptoms will usually result.

3. *Arteriosclerosis* — occurs at an advanced age, tinnitus is present, hearing loss is usually bilateral, and other symptoms and signs of generalized arteriosclerosis are present.

4. *Cholesteotoma* — a history of previous ear infections with mastoiditis is usually obtained. X-ray will show the lesion and there is a history of unilateral hearing reduction.

5. *Wax in ear canal* — a history of wax accumulating in the ears with frequent cleaning out of the canals.

6. *Upper respiratory infections* — history of colds, sore throats, earaches, sinusitis, etc.

HEAD INJURIES

Questions

When did you have a head injury? How did it happen? What part of the head was injured? Were you unconscious, how long? Did you know where you were when you woke up? Did you lose your memory for what happened just before the accident and after the accident? Did you have bleeding from the nose, the ears or the mouth? How long were you in the hospital and how long were you kept in bed after the accident? Did the doctors tell you that you had a fractured skull?

Interpretation

Unconsciousness or bleeding from the cranial orifices means that the brain was damaged seriously. The greater the span of memory loss before and after the accident, the greater the brain damage. At times, a light blow to the head will produce serious brain damage with serious symptoms. Contrecoup brain damage may occur in that the brain will be damaged on the side opposite the head injury. Was there a period of clear consciousness after the accident and then unconsciousness (middle meningeal artery rupture)? How long did you have headache after the accident? What was the state of your nerves following the accident? (A measure of emotional stability following a head accident). A few weeks or months following the accident did you have increasing headache with weakness of an arm or leg or some trouble in feeling things on one side of the body? (subdural hematoma).

Facial Pains

Questions

Ever had facial neuralgia or tic douloureux or other pains in the face? Did any actions bring on the facial pains such as chewing, swallowing, scratching, itching, yawning, etc.? Did you have any infected teeth or sinus infection at the time?

Interpretations

1. *Trigeminal neuralgia or tic douloureux* — occurs in middle or late life, is sudden in onset, usually triggered by certain stimuli as chewing, swallowing, rubbing the face, yawning, brushing the teeth, etc. Pain is very intense, located in one or more of the divisions of the trigeminal nerve, responds to very few medicines.

2. *Atypical facial neuralgia* — occurs at any age, usually not acute in onset, not so intense pain, more like a dullness, a throbbing, a waving sensation, or it is described by many other different adjectives, usually bizarre. It is not confined to any anatomic division of the fifth nerve. The personality is usually unstable with much emotional overlay of symptoms. It may be helped by many and varied medicinal, suggestive and physiotherapeutic measures.

3. *Facial pain* — a constant pain in one side of the face must be checked for the presence of dental, sinus, mouth, throat, nose, neck, and ear conditions, or temporomandibular joint conditions.

Teeth Conditions

Inquire about the care of the teeth, dentures, fillings, abscesses, wisdom teeth, why teeth were pulled (one hears of many varied reasons from patients as to why their teeth are pulled and these may prove to be clues to other problems.

Neck Conditions

Questions

Any trouble with your arms during your life, any pains, any numbness and tingling, any difference in the size of your arms, any weakness in the arms or hands, any change of color, any sweating of the palms of the hands, have the finger nails changed at all recently?

Interpretation

1. *Brachial neuritis* — pain in the shoulder and scapular area, down the arm, numbness and tingling in the arm and fingers, tender areas around the shoulder joints, limitation of motion due to pain, usually unilateral but may be bilateral, takes many weeks to recover, responds slowly to physical therapy and vitamin B_{12} injections.

2. *Cervical rib* — pain, numbness, tingling, sensory and motor disturbances in arm often bilateral, positive x-ray.

3. *Scalenus anticus syndrome* — symptoms simulate cervical rib.

4. *Spinal cord pathology* — viz:

a. *Subacute combined sclerosis* — may precede the blood findings of pernicious anemia, presenting usually numbness and tingling in the hands and feet with disturbances of deep sensations showing up in difficulty in walking, in placing the feet where one wants them to be placed, in stiffness of the joints, weakness of the arms and legs and possibly dragging of the toe due to pyramidal tract involvement and some incoordination of the hands and fingers.

b. *Spinal cord neoplasm* — a progression of symptoms of weakness, stiffness, walking difficulties, arms and hand difficulties, sensation disturbances, pains, bladder and bowel symptoms, and occasionally atrophy of muscles of the hand and legs. All these symptoms bespeak pressure and irritation of the various ascending and descending nervous pathways in the spinal cord and on nerve cells.

c. *Amyotrophic lateral sclerosis* — progressive weakness of the arms and legs with fibrillary twitchings of the muscles of the arms and legs associated with increasing stiffness of the legs and walking difficulties — all due to involvement of the pyramidal tracts and the anterior horn nerve cells — occurring usually in persons in middle life and older.

d. *Progressive muscular atrophy* — progressive weakness of the legs and arms associated with fibrillary twitchings of the muscles occurring in persons of middle or older life, all due to involvement of the anterior horn cells — a chronic, progressive, deteriorating, neurologic disease.

e. *Multiple sclerosis* — progressive stiffness and weakness of one or both arms and legs with coordination difficulties such as trouble in placing the feet and hands where the individual wishes to place them, difficulty in writing, picking up objects, bladder and bowel symptoms, numbness or prickling sensations in the arms and legs occurring in persons usually under the age of 40 years. Visual and cerebellar symptoms may also be present.

f. *Tabes dorsalis* — due to syphilitic involvement of the central nervous system and usually causing symptoms of ataxia in the arms and legs, all due to the involvement of the posterior columns of the spinal cord resulting in deep sensory disturbances, along with bladder and bowel disturbances, visual difficulties of optic atrophy, pupillary disturbances and other somatic complaints.

LEGS

Questions

Any pains or numbness, pins and needles in the legs, any trouble walking or in putting your feet where you want to put them, any trouble walking in the dark, do you limp on one leg, do you drag your feet or stumble, do you wear out the toe of one shoe more than the other while walking, have you had any cramps in the leg muscles, any twitchings of the muscles, is any one leg smaller than the other, any varicose veins, do your legs jump at times?

Interpretation

1. *Sciatic neuritis* — pain in the back of the thigh, the knee, and the lower leg radiating from the hip or the low back accompanied by hypalgesia and hypesthesia, varying degrees of weakness and a limp from favoring the leg. History of a back injury or strain or an infection prior to the onset of the neuritis.

2. *Spinal cord pathology* — viz.:

    a. *Subacute combined sclerosis* — see above in section on the arm.

    b. *Spinal cord neoplasm* — see above in section on the arm.

    c. *Amyotrophic lateral sclerosis* — see above in section on the arm.

    d. *Progressive muscular atrophy* — see above in section on the arm.

    e. *Multiple sclerosis* — see above in the section on the arm.

    f. *Tabes dorsalis* — see above in the section on the arm.

GENERAL QUESTIONS

Inquire also about the following in taking a neurologic history:

1. Fractures.
2. Accidents.
3. Residuals of accidents.
4. Hospitalizations associated with accidents.
5. Litigation results.
6. Operations.
7. General medical conditions such as diseases of heart, lungs, thyroid, liver, intestines, kidneys, stomach, genitals, bladder, skin, diabetes, vomiting.
8. Fevers such as: typhoid, scarlet, rheumatic, malaria, encephalitis, sleeping sickness.
9. Allergy exhibiting itself as asthma, hay fever, hives.
10. Tobacco habits.
11. Alcohol or drug habits.
12. Venereal diseases.
13. Childhood habits.
14. Birth injuries.
15. Emotional or mental troubles.

In any neurologic or psychiatric problem, one should always ask about the sexual function. With men, one can ask directly about the ability to produce an erection, etc. With women one should ask sexual questions more carefully, beginning with a history of her menstrual life and leading to sexual desires of late and any possible difficulties of late.

SUMMARY OF NEUROLOGIC HISTORY REMINDERS

Have You Ever Had:

1. Headache — migraine.
2. Tender spots on your head.
3. Bumps on your head.
4. Injuries to your head — hit your head — any bleeding from your nose, ears, mouth — any trouble with headaches, dizziness since the accident.
5. Unconsciousness — been knocked out — dazed — confused — how long.
6. Convulsions — fits, epilepsy (other terms used by patients — dizzy, weak spells, etc.) Any one in your family with spells?
7. Dizziness.
8. Eye troubles—double vision—poor vision—blurred vision—glasses.
9. Ear troubles — hearing difficulty — ringing in the ears — operations of the ears.
10. Throat troubles — swallowing difficulties — lump in the throat.
11. Teeth troubles.
12. Facial pains — paralysis — neuralgia.
13. Neck troubles — injuries — pains — aches — spasms.
14. Shoulder troubles — pains — aches — weakness — fractures.
15. Arm troubles — pains — neuritis — neuralgia — weakness — injuries — fractures — numbness — stiffness.
16. Tremors of the hands — fingers — shakings — tremblings — stiffness — color change.
17. Leg troubles — pains — neuritis — neuralgia — weakness — numbness — cramps — fractures — limitation of motion.
18. Back trouble — pain-limitation of motion — weakness — injuries — catches in the back — cramps.
19. Walking troubles — staggering — stiffness — tripping — walking in the dark — weakness.
20. Urinary troubles — starting and stopping the stream — urgency·— losing the urine.
21. Erection trouble.
22. St. Vitus dance — chorea — influenza — encephalitis — or sleeping sickness — brain fever.
23. Polio — paralysis of any kind.
24. Neuritis — neuralgia — rheumatism — sciatica or pains anywhere.
25. Fevers of any kind — scarlet fever — rheumatic fever — malaria fever — typhoid fever.
26. Allergies — hay fever — asthma — hives.
27. Nervous breakdowns — mental illness — been in any mental hospital.
28. Operations — accidents.
29. Sleep troubles.
30. A stroke.

3. *Neurologic Examination Reminders*

THE AUTHOR WAS TAUGHT to begin the neurologic examination with the head and to finish with the toes. In this method, one examines each anatomical part completely for abnormality of the functioning of the central nervous system, peripheral nervous system and the autonomic nervous system. As one moves down the body, one may incorporate in the neurologic examination the important aspects of a general physical examination. After one has developed a method, one must discipline oneself constantly and severely so as not to leave this or that aspect out of the examination as the days and the examinations go by. Occasionally, for lack of time one is tempted to leave·a certain test out of the examination. If this procedure continues, one ends up inevitably with a very brief and superficial neurologic examination. For instance, if one were to leave out the examination of the optic fundus because it takes time, or to leave out the tests for testing deep sensation, one would soon miss diagnoses. If time is short, it is far better to have the patient return and finish the examination the next time.

One needs the following tools for a complete, practical neurologic examination, which can be done in the office of any company or at the bedside in the company's dispensary or at the patient's home. More elaborate neurologic methods call for more elaborate tools, available only at neurologic centers. I want to keep this examination practical for the average occupational physician. The tools are as follows:

1. stethoscope.
2. blood pressure apparatus.
3. safety pin.
4. ophthalmoscope.
5. otoscopic attachment for the ophthalmoscope.
6. tuning fork (128 vibrations to the second).
7. a wisp of cotton or the edge of one's coat pocket handkerchief would do.
8. 2 small metal tubes with tops that screw on tightly to keep hot and cold water intact.
9. reflex hammer.

10. tape measure of a steel type which recoils easily into the round metal container.

11. wooden tongue blades.

The tools can be carried easily in a small leather bag. A Snell Visual Acuity chart is usually in place on the wall of an occupational medical office and the physician usually wears a watch of some type.

At the end of this chapter, I have listed a summary of the Neurologic Examination Tests.

Preparation of the Patient for the Neurologic Examination

Men: Have patient undress leaving shorts on. The nurse, if available, may be called to take notes dictated by the examining physician during the examination.

Women: Have the nurse assist the patient in undressing, leaving the underpants on and draping the patient with suitable garments. The nurse should remain during the examination. She may take notes dictated by the physician during the examination. During the examination the woman should be exposed only during the examination of the particular area of the body which is being examined at that time.

General Appearance

With the patient standing with their feet on the floor, look for any deformities. Notice the posture, the stance, the skin condition. Look for a tilt of the head, the position of the shoulders, the general body development, for local atrophy. Notice the nutritional state; whether sweating is present. Look for tendon contractures, scars, facial expressions. Observe the emotional state. Look for abnormal attitudes that might be a diagnostic clue, such flexion of the fingers, wrist and elbows on one side, suggesting hemiplegia, or the masking of the facial expression with generalized rigidity and flexion of the head, trunk, fingers, elbows, and knees suggesting Parkinsonism. One should learn to observe well as more diagnoses are missed by *"not looking rather than by not knowing."*

NEUROLOGIC EXAMINATION

Test	Testing	For
1. Stand here toes, heels together (barefeet). Eyes open, then closed.	Position sense Romberg Posterior column Peripheral nerves	Ataxia; tabes; multiple sclerosis, pernicious anemia with subacute combined sclerosis, cerebellar disturbance, malingering; hysteria

2. Open eyes, stand on right foot—now left. Close eyes and repeat.

Coordination, equilibrium, strength, (in cerebellar diseases, patient sways with eyes open or closed).

Above disorders plus dystonia

3. Jump up and down on right foot—now left foot.

Same as above plus rigidity and spasticity.

Same as above plus Parkinsonism and hemiparesis

4. Walk naturally across room and back again.

Same as number 3 plus gait, associated arm motions, posture, muscle status.

Ataxia; atrophy, dystrophy; dystonia; Parkinsonism; limps; spastic gait; old polio; hemiplegia; painful calluses

5. Walk heel to toe in a straight line across the room.

Equilibrium

Ataxia; multiple sclerosis; subacute combined sclerosis; tabes

6. Walk on toes—now on heels.

Same as above plus strength of leg muscles.

Foot drop; polio residuals; fracture residuals; ataxia and above disorders

7. Walk sidewise to the right then to the left.

Spasticity, rigidity, ataxia (hemiplegic foot will drag; a Parkinson's leg will be stiff and slow.)

Hemiplegia; Parkinsonism; ataxia

8. Squat down to the floor.

Balance, motor strength, spasticity and rigidity.

Same as number 3

9. (1) Listen to head with stethoscope
(2) Run fingers over head
(3) Percuss head

(1) Vascular noises
(2) Bumps of skull and scalp.
(3) Tenderness

(1) Vascular lesions; angioma; aneurysm
(2) Bony erosions from brain tumors; wens; cysts
(3) Bony disease or injury

10. Examine scalp with pin.

Sensory intergrity for pain

Expanding intracranial lesion as tumor, abscess, hematoma,

Test	Testing	For
		cerebral hemorrhage or thrombosis, hysteria
11. (1) Place tuning fork on top of head. Ask patient "Where do you feel it?" (Weber test)	(1) Integrity of middle ear and external auditory canal. In middle ear or external auditory canal disease, lateralization occurs on affected side. Normally, the sound is heard equally on both sides.	(1) Lesions of middle ear and external auditory canal
(2) Place tuning fork on mastoid process. Ask patient "tell me when you do not feel the fork buzzing." At that point, place tuning fork in front of ear and ask, "Do you hear the tuning fork?" (Rinne Test)	(2) Integrity of air conduction system. In middle ear diseases, bone conduction is greater than air conduction—in nerve deafness, air conduction is superior unless hearing is markedly affected	(2) Middle ear disease nerve deafness
12. Examine eyes (1) General appearance	(1) Condition of sclerae, conjunctivae, corneae and lids.	(1) Icteric sclerae Inflamed sclerae, conjunctivitis; corneal scars; opacities; blepharitis
	(2) Position of eyeballs.	(2) Strabismus Exophthalmos
	(3) Nystagmus	(3) *Type of nystagmus:* congenital nystagmus; occupational . nystagmus; nystagmus in diseases such as multiple sclerosis; brain tumors; encephalitis; etc.
(2) Ocular tension test: Place index	(2) Increased intraocular tension	(2) Glaucoma

fingers gently over eyeball and alternately push and relax these fingers over the eyeball. One soon learns the feel of normal tension and will recognize abnormal tension readily

(3) Listen to eyes with stethoscope

(3) Vascular bruit noises

(3) Vascular lesions such as aneurysm at base of brain around circle of Willis

(4) Apply a wisp of cotton to the lateral edges of the corneae with the patient looking to the opposite direction. Patient with normal cornea will blink quickly.

(4) Corneal reflex Integrity of cornea and corneal reflex nerve pathway

(4) Lesions of cornea; trigeminal and facial nerves and of brain stem

(5) Extraocular movements: Follow my finger upward

(5) Ocular motions and muscle coordination (Ocular nerves and muscles)

(5) Ocular muscle weaknesses from lesions of brain stem; base of brain; orbit, frontal skull area and increased intracranial pressure

(6) Look ahead. I'll put a light near your eyes. (in a darkened room)

(6) Pupillary action, size, shape, direct and consensual light reflex

(6) Brain tumor and abscesses, encephalitis; neurosyphilis; meningitis; brain injuries; subdural hematoma or thrombosis. Local eye conditions as iridectomy; eye injuries, etc. Hornor's syndrome Argyll-Robertson pupils

Test	Testing	For
(7) Look a little to the left. (Examine right fundus.) Look a little to the right. (Examine left fundus)	(7) Condition of media, lens, fundus retinal blood vessels	(7) Opacities of media and lens. Optic disc conditions as atrophy; choking from brain tumor; Multiple Sclerosis; optic neuritis and retrobulbar neuritis. Retinal diseases as hemorrhage; exudates; congenital defects; arteriosclerosis; hypertension. Metabolic diseases such as diabetes; nephritis; and degenerate diseases
(8) Look at the light and tell me if you see double. (Hold light in all directions around eyes)	(8) Diplopia, integrity of ocular muscles	(8) Brain tumor; abscess; encephalitis; multiple sclerosis; tabes; virus diseases
(9) As examiner faces patient, cover patient's right eye with your left hand. Test nasal field of left eye by bringing wiggling fingers of your right hand forward in from patient's right side until he says he sees the fingers. Cover patient's left eye with your left hand and repeat test for nasal field of right eye. Test temporal visual field of each eye by bringing your wiggling fingers in from patient's right and left side until he sees them.	(9) Visual fields (gross). Hemianopsia and quadrantanopsia may develop by brain lesions	(9) Brain tumors; abscesses; multiple sclerosis; optic neuritis; retrobulbar neuritis

(10) Have patient stand twenty feet away from a Snellen's test chart. The letters of the top line are usually seen at a distance of 200 feet and those at the bottom at 20 feet. The lines in between are visible at 30, 40, 50, 70 and 100 feet. The person with normal vision reads the lowest line and his vision is recorded as 20/20. If one can read the top line only, his vision is recorded as 20/200. What is the lowest line of letters that you can read with your right eye without glasses? (Have patient cover his left eye by *cupping* his left hand over the left eye.) Now read with your left eye (cup your right hand over your right eye). Test both eyes with glasses for correction reading

(10) Visual acuity. Integrity of ocular system of vision from the cornea to the occipital cortex

(10) Lesions of: cornea; vitreous; retina; optic nerve; optic tract; optic chiasm; optic radiation; occipital cortex; superior colliculus. From: traumatic, toxic, inflammatory, infectious, degenerative, neoplastic, metabolic, conditions

13. Wrinkle your forehead up, frown, close your eyes, show your teeth, sniff and move your nostrils in and out. (Dilate and contract your nasal fossae.) Blow out your cheeks, purse your lips, whistle, pull your ears back.

Facial nerve

Bell's palsy (peripheral paralysis). *Facial paralysis* (central paralysis)—usually associated with a hemiplegia from a vascular or neoplastic condition. *Thalamic facial weakness.* Present only when patient laughs, smiles

Test	Testing	For
		or cries. *Cortical irritation* as tonic or clonic spasms. *Habit and reflex spasms* of face. Blephorospasms; tics; grimaces; chorea —athetotic motions
14. Put out your tongue. I want to test your taste. Keep your tongue out during the test and signal with your hand when you identify the taste. (Test with sweet, sour, salty and bitter solutions in this order.) At best, this is not a satisfactory test	Sensory taste fibers of facial nerve which supply the anterior two-thirds of the tongue	Facial nerve lesions and their location— whether in front of the facial canal, in the canal, or intracranially. If taste is lost lesion is in facial canal
15. Bite hard against your teeth. (Palpate action of masseter and temporal muscles on both sides.) Bite hard on this tongue blade. (Hold tongue blade between teeth on each side and note the depths of the bite in the blade on each side.	Trigeminal motor nerve. The masseter and temporal muscles. *In peripheral lesions* motor root is paralyzed. Patient can't move point of jaw to affected side. Jaw deviates to affected side. No muscular contraction of masseter and temporal muscles when biting motions are attempted. Fibrillations and atrophy are present. In *brain stem lesions* unilateral or bilateral motor paralysis may occur. *In cortical and pyramidal tract lesions,* usually no paralysis as motor	*Peripheral lesions* as neuritis; tumors; basilar skull fracture; meningitis; stab wounds, *brain stem* lesions—as encephalitis; degenerations; syphilis; syringomyelia and progressive muscular atrophy; hemorrhage. *Cortical and Pyramidal tract lesions* as tumors; hemorrhage

nucleus has bilateral
innervation

Observe masticatory
muscles for abnormal
involuntary muscle
actions

Clonic or tonic spasms.
Rhythmic contraction

Cortical lesions pro-
ducing *Jacksonian
convulsions*; clonic or
tonic.
Paralysis agitans—
rhythmic

16. Using a pinpoint,
test forehead and face,
and rest of scalp, first
one side and then the
other. Do you feel
this? Does it seem
sharp or dull? Is
there any difference
in feeling between the
two sides?

Painful sensation of tri-
geminal sensory fibers
Analgesia or hypal-
gesia will result from
paralytic lesions and
hyperalgesia and pain
from irritative lesions

Peripheral lesions—from
gasserian ganglion to
face and forehead, as
basilar meningitis and
skull fractures;
tumors; and bony
disease around exit
foramina of nerves
leaving skull

Psychogenic sensory
disturbances end at
midline while organic
disturbances run over
midline

*Gasserian ganglion
lesions*—tumors, in-
flammatory

Using a wisp of cotton
or a corner of a pocket
handkerchief, test
forehead and face. Do
you feel this on both
sides? Is there any
difference? Close your
eyes and tell me where
I am touching you.
Using a tube of hot
water and a tube of
cold water, test fore-
head and face.

Light touch sensations
of trigeminal sensory
fibers. Diminished
light touch sensation
(hypesthesia) results
from paralytic lesions.
Increased sensation
from irritative lesions.
(Hyperesthesia.)
Thermal sensation of
trigeminal sensory
fibers

Sensory root lesions
from exit from the
pons to gasserian
ganglion; tumors;
meningitis; neuritis;
hemorrhage; trauma

Brain stem lesions
causing onion skin
representation of
sensory disturbance.
Lower lesions of
spinal descending
tract or upper
cervical cord and
lower brain stem pro-
duce sensory disturb-
ances around
the nose.

Test	*Testing*	*For*
		Higher lesions produce wider concentric or circular areas of facial sensory disturbance, such as vascular, tumors, encephalitis, syphilis, multiple sclerosis, syringobulbia
17. Observe face for any change in facial skin color, skin texture, skin dryness or wetness or atrophy of facial tissues.	Vasomotor, secretory and trophic functions	Facial hemiatrophy; progressive facial hemiatrophy; emotional conditions
18. Open your mouth and say, "Ah." Hold tongue down with tongue depressor and note position and movement of uvula.	Integrity of ninth and tenth (glossopharyngeal and Vagus) nerves. Since these nerves are so closely related anatomically and functionally, they are usually studied and tested together. In paralysis or weakness of uvula, uvula will be raised upwards to opposite sides on saying "Ah." Swallowing of liquids may be difficult.	*Supranuclear lesions:* Pseudobulbar palsy: lesions between cortex and brain stem, i.e., vascular, encephalitis, multiple sclerosis, Parkinsonism
Touch the posterior wall of the pharynx with the tongue depressor and pinpoint.	Pharyngeal sensation and reaction. No pharyngeal contraction and no gagging results from lesions of ninth and tenth nerves	Brain stem—(nuclear) multiple sclerosis; acute anterior poliomyelitis; Landry's paralysis; epidemic encephalitis; amyotrophic lateral sclerosis; syringo-

		myelia, progressive muscular atrophy
19. Note quality of voice	Contraction of vocal cords Recurrent laryngeal nerve	Aortic aneurism; brain stem lesions; mediastinal tumors; apical tuberculosis; dilation of left auricle; enlarged neck glands.
Place mirror in pharynx to examine vocal cords. (or refer to a specialist)	Speech is nasal and difficult to understand. Swallowing and mastication difficult.	*Peripheral*; hemorrhage; basilar skull disease; meningitis; tumors; multiple neuritis from lead; alcohol; arsenic and diphtheritic conditions
	Integrity of vagus trunk. In deep neck operations the vagus trunk may be injured causing: unilateral paralysis and anesthesia of soft palate, pharynx and larynx; gastric dilatation and pain, vomiting, loss of thirst and hunger; loss of ipsilateral oculocardiac reflex. When both vagus trunks are involved death occurs through cardiac and respiratory failure	*Vagus trunk lesions.* Glossopharyngeal neuralgia vasovagal attacks. Spasms of pharynx; larynx; tongue and esophagus in tetany; hysteria; tabes; hydrophobia and reflex from digestive and respiratory conditions Vagotonia; including motion sickness; pseudoanginal attacks; high sugar tolerance spastic bowel; gastric hyperacidity
20. Rotate your head to the right (against resistance of examiner's left hand held against chin) Rotate your head to the left	Integrity of spinal accessory nerve and sternocleidomastoid muscles. Each muscle pulls chin to opposite side. Paralysis, atrophy, fibrillations, inability to rotate chin	*Peripheral lesions*; meningitis; hemorrhage; tumors; basilar skull injuries: basilar skull disease; exudates; surgical neck operations

Test	Testing	For
With free hand test the sternocleidomastoid muscle for contractile power		*Brain stem (nuclear) lesions: amyotrophic* lateral sclerosis; progressive muscular
Shrug your shoulders up and down (with and without resistance)	Integrity and strength of trapezii muscles. Paralysis-atrophy, fibrillations, inability to shrug shoulders	atrophy; myelitis; acute anterior poliomyelitis; syringobulbia and syringomyelia. Supranuclear (cortical and pyramidal tract) lesions: usually no symptoms because of bilateral cortical innervation of nuclear spinal accessory nerve
Observe for abnormal involuntary motions of neck	Presence of spasmodic torticollis. Spasm of muscle which rotates head to opposite side	Torticollis (wry neck). Not a disease of spinal accessory nerve; but it involves muscles supplied by it: irritative labrynth lesions; occupational conditions in which head is tilted to one side; toxic or infectious, congenital; psychogenic (emotional)
21. Stick out your tongue. Raise it, lower it and move it from side to side	Integrity of hypoglossal nerve (twelfth cranial nerve) and of tongue muscles. Atrophy fibrillations and weakness of tongue on side of lesion in peripheral lesions. On opposite side of lesion in brain stem or nuclear lesions and in cortical	*Peripheral lesions (infranuclear):* meningitis; trauma; neoplasms; at base of skull; basilar skull diseases; aneurysm of vertebral artery and internal carotid; fractures and diseases of base of skull; stab wounds; inflammatory

and internal capsule lesions

and neoplastic lesions of neck. Fractured dislocation of atlas. *Brain Stem (nuclear) Lesions:* The hypoglossal nucleus is usually involved with other medullary motor nuclei and the condition is known as bulbar palsy (marked difficulty in phonation, mastication, speaking and swallowing)

Progressive muscular atrophy; amyotrophic lateral sclerosis syringobulbia; Landry's paralysis; multiple sclerosis; acute encephalitis; syphilis, vascular lesions, neoplastic lesion

Cortical and Internal Capsule Lesions (Supranuclear): Vascular—hemorrhage, thrombosis. or embolism; *Degenerative*, inflammatory, neoplastic

Observe tongue for gross involuntary abnormal motions

Condition and state of tongue—involuntary motions of tongue associated with noises

Emotional causes: and accompanying signs of hysteria

22. Let me see your neck. (Examine for thyroid, lymph glands, tumors, asymmetry, atrophies, hyper-

Neck abnormalities. Muscles of neck and shoulders

Thyroid disease; lymph adenopathy; atrophies; hypertrophies; varicosities; limitation of motion

Test	*Testing*	*For*
trophies, etc. of neck and shoulder area). Move your neck forward, backward, to the left and right (with and without resistance)		
Can you feel this pin? Is there any difference in feeling between the two sides of the neck? Can you feel this light touch? (Touch with a wisp of cotton) Does this feel warm or cold to you? (Test with hot and cold tubes.)	Sensation of neck	Sensory disturbances associated with cortical, internal capsule, brain stem and peripheral lesions of cranial nerves
23. (Use your own resistance to test fingers, wrists, arms and shoulders.)		
(1) Put your arms out straight in front of you and spread your fingers wide apart	(1) Motor strength of movements, rigidity, spasticity, and coordination of shoulders, arm, and finger muscles. Atrophy, fibrillations, color, skin condition	(1-2) Motor weakness; sensory disturbances; vasomotor disturbances; as: hemiparesis; peripheral neuritis; amyotrophic lateral sclerosis; progressive muscular atrophy; progressive muscular dystrophy; syringomyelia
(2) Hold your fingers tight together Grip my hands Hold your fingers out straight (try to flex fingers) Make a fist (flexion of fingers)	(2) Abduction, adduction, flexion, extension	

Cock your wrists up—
down
Bend your elbows up
tightly
Straighten out your
arms
Raise your arms side-
wise, and over your
shoulder.
Shrug your shoulders
up

(3) Grip my hands—
hard—let go quickly
(repeat this)

(3) Strength, coordina-
tion, muscle tone, ease
of relaxing

(3) Myotonia congenita
or acquisita; motor
weakness; spasticity;
rigidity; atrophic
diseases; spinal cord
diseases; rupture of
intervertebral disc

24. Rotate your forearms
back and forth like
this (alternating
pronation and supin-
ation)

Strength of pronators
and supinators—and
alternate motion rate

Muscle diseases; coor-
dination diseases;
Parkinsonism; spastic
conditions

25. With your eyes open,
slowly put the tip of
your index finger on
your nose. Now do it
with your eyes closed

Integrity of posterior
columns of spinal cord
and of cerebellar
pathways. Nonequil-
ibratory ataxia

Multiple sclerosis; tabes
dorsalis; subacute
combined sclerosis;
cerebellar lesions

26. Hold your right arm
out (then left arm
later on). I am going
to test you with this
pin (start on outer
side of arm near
shoulder and come
down to the fingers—
then test up the inner
side of the arm after
testing the hand.
Compare the two
sides) *Does it feel*

Painful sensation from
higher cervical cord
segments to higher
thoracic segments.
Hypalgesia, hyperal-
gesia

Peripheral and central
lesions, as brachial
neuritis; pressure
neuropathy such as
ulnar neuropathy,
multiple neuritis;
central lesions as
spinal cord lesions

Test	Testing	For
sharp? Does it feel dull anywhere? Is there any difference between the two sides?		
If a dull area is found, map it out by testing from the dull area to the normal area and outline dull area with a fountain pen or skin pencil. *Can you tell the difference between the sharp point and the dull end of the pin?*	Hypalgesia will be present in conditions which destroy pain sensation as hemorrhage around central canal spinal cord neoplasm, syringomyelia. Hyperalgesia may be present in tabes, herpes zoster radiculitis; and hypertrophic spinal arthritis	Rupture of intervertebral disc; cervical arthritis; syringomyelia; cortical lesions as tumors; internal capsule lesions; herpes zoster; radiculitis; and brain tumors
27. Hold your right arm out—then the left arm later. I shall test you with this piece of cotton. (Proceed in the same fashion as with the pin)	Tactile sensation	Same as conditions in #26
28. For hysteria—close your eyes and tell me where I am touching you. For testing of hysterical analgesia, use the "yes-no" test. Use the wisp of cotton. The orders to the patient will be as follows: Close your eyes and say "yes" when I touch you and "no" when I don't. Stroke the normal area first, several times and the patient	Hysterical analgesia If the patient has a positive test, it means that the sensory stimulus is reaching consciousness	Conversion hysteria

will say "yes" each
time you stroke him.
Then shift to the
alleged area of re-
duced sensation. The
patient, if hysterical,
will usually say with
each stroke, "no."

29. Hold your right arm   Thermal sensation   Same as conditions
    out—then your left   in #26
    arm later. I shall test
    you with these hot and
    cold tubes. Tell me if
    it feels hot or cold.
    Compare two sides

30. Hold out your right   Deep sensation.   Tabes dorsalis; multiple
    arm—then left arm   Vibratory sensation   sclerosis; subacute
    later. I shall put this   through posterior   combined sclerosis;
    tuning fork on certain   columns of spinal   peripheral neuritis;
    spots of your arm and   cord.   spinal cord tumors;
    shoulder. (Periosteal   Cortical sensation.   Friedreich's ataxia.
    surfaces as shoulder   Integrity of   Brain tumors and
    point, clavicles,   peripheral nerves   abscesses; subdural
    sternum.) Tell me   hematoma
    when you don't feel
    it buzzing anymore.
    Measure duration in
    seconds

31. Let me have one of   Deep sensation. Two-   See #30
    your fingers. I shall   point discrimination.
    put two pins on your   Cortical sensibility
    finger and with your   Normally, two points
    eyes closed please tell   can be recognized at
    me whether you feel   2-3 mm. on tips of
    one or two pins.   fingers. In disease, a
    (Move pins away and   greater distance be-
    towards each other   tween points is
    until patient identifies   necessary before two
    whether one or two   points are recognized
    pins are on the finger.
    Note the distance.)

Test	Testing	For
32. Close your eyes. I shall move your finger up or down. Tell me which way I am moving it. (Grasp finger on sides.)	Deep sensation Position sense (cortical sensation) Normally a person can detect very slight movements. In disease of deep sensory pathways, the patient cannot tell accurately if it is being moved and/or in what direction	See #30 In aged and arthritic patients position sense may be altered without any nerve pathology
33. With your eyes closed, I shall place different sized and shaped objects in your hand. I want you to describe the object to me	Stereognosis-cortical sensation (parietal). The ability to recognize the size and form of an object by palpation	Parietal lobe; cortex lesions as tumors, abscesses; vascular lesions
34. Sit in your chair (or on the bed). I want to look at your arms and shoulders (examine for atrophy of muscles or muscle groups)	Integrity of anterior horn cell and peripheral motor nerve	Amyotrophic lateral sclerosis; progressive muscular atrophy; syringomyelia; Acute and chronic poliomyelitis; spinal cord tumors; hypertrophic spinal arthritis; peripheral nerve lesions (toxic, infectious, traumatic) atrophy from disuse; as in hemiplegia
35. Examine for hypertrophy	Integrity of muscular structure. Hypertrophic muscles are weaker due to fibrotic and cellular changes	Progressive muscular dystrophy

36. Examine for fibril-
    lary twitchings.
    Tapping a muscle
    with a percussion
    hammer may initiate
    fibrillary twitchings.
    Fibrillary twitchings
    are slow or rapid
    contractions of indiv-
    idual muscle fibers or
    bundle of fibers. One
    must be patient in
    looking for twitchings.
    Room temperature
    may influence them.
    *Joints are not moved
    by fibrillary twitchings*

Fibrillary twitchings
Integrity of anterior
horn cells and peri-
pheral nerve lesions

Amyotrophic lateral
sclerosis; progressive
muscular atrophy;
syringomyelia; bulbar
palsies; herniated
disc pressure

37. I want to do some
    tests on your arm—so
    just relax. Alternately
    flex and extend the
    elbow. Then the wrist
    and the fingers. Com-
    pare tension of
    muscles in both arms.
    Normally the elbow,
    wrists, and fingers
    should move easily
    with no resistance
    felt by the examiner.
    In hypotonia the
    joints move more
    freely than normal.
    In hypertonia, they
    move less freely

Muscle tone
Integrity of neural
pathways preserving
muscle tone

Hypotonicity: Acute
and chronic polio-
myelitis; tabes
dorsalis; progressive
muscular atrophy;
amyotonia congenita;
cerebellar disease
(ipsilateral); amyo-
trophic lateral
sclerosis (if anterior-
horn disease is more
advanced than
pyramidal tract
disease)
Hypertonicity: Hemi-
plegia; monoplegia;
quadriplegia due to
vascular lesions;
neoplasms; abscesses
and other space-
occupying cerebral
lesions; Parkinson-

Test	*Testing*	*For*
		ism; multiple sclerosis; amyotrophic lateral sclerosis; subacute combined sclerosis; spinal cord tumors and other space-occupying spinal lesions; herniated disc and hypertrophic arthritis
38. With a percussion hammer, stimulate muscles	Irritability of muscles	Pyramidal tract disease Tetany
39. Palpate muscles with your hand	Muscle consistency. Pain may be present in myositis	Myositis; myofibrositis; progressive muscular dystrophy; (will show hard rubber consistency); Hypotonia (will show a softness)
40. Observe shoulders and arms for *tremors.* Be patient and observe patient at different times. Tremors are affected by emotions, attention, rest, motion, room temperature, and muscular activity	Integrity of neuro-muscular mechanism	*Coarse tremors:* Psychoneurosis, striatal disease as Parkinsonism; progressive lenticular degeneration; cerebellar and mid brain disease *Fine tremors:* Psychoneurosis; hyperthyroidism; alcoholism; toxic states; general paresis; rhythmical tremor; Parkinsonism; intention tremor. multiple sclerosis—coarse and irregular —voluntary senile tremors; posthemiplegic tremors

41. Observe body for *choreiform motions*—involuntary, irregular in rate, rhythm, amplitude and force. Worse from attention, emotion, or voluntary motions, seemingly purposeless. At times, they may be minimal. Observations of nurses and others over the 24 hours are important

Choreiform movements, integrity of lenticular nucleus

Sydenham's chorea (children); Huntington's chorea (adults); chronic progressive chorea; epidemic encephalitis; vascular lesions in basal ganglia. Hysteria

42. Observe body for *athetotic movements.* Slow, purposeless, irregular, writhing, sinuous, twisting movements involving preferably fingers and toes but at times face, limbs and neck muscles. Facial grimacing does occur when face is involved

Athetosis. Integrity of corpus striatum

Congenital athetosis: Degenerative athetosis in early childhood and adolescence

43. Observe body for habit and reflex spasms

Habit and reflex spasms. Integrity of neuromuscular mechanism and possible presence of emotional difficulties

Blepharospasm (emotional). Spasmodic torticollis (emotional or corpus striatum)
Tics (emotional or early dystonia musculorum deformans)
Reflex spasms:
  1. Tic douloureux
  2. Hamstrings (sciatic neuritis)
  3. Dental conditions
  4. Hemifacial spasms from:
    a. Trigeminal nerve disease

Test	*Testing*	*For*
		b. Cortical irritation (Jacksonian convulsion)
		c. Facial nerve irritation
		d. No obvious pathology
		5. Arms and legs in pyramidal tract disease
44. Observe body for dystonia. Large, slow exaggerated athetoid movements causing body tension.	Dystonia. Integrity of corpus striatum	Dystonia musculorum deformans
45. Observe convulsion if one occurs and postconvulsive state (drowsiness and sleepiness in generalized convulsions—weakness of part affected in Jacksonian convulsions)	Convulsions. For source of irritative cause of convulsions (sensory or motor)	*Generalized convulsions:* 1. Idiopathic epilepsy 2. Neoplasm; abscesses; subdural hematoma; encephalitis; vascular lesions; cerebral atrophy; general paresis; infections of central nervous system and meninges; infectious diseases; allergy; hysteria (not typical) *Jacksonian convulsion:* Neoplasm; abscess; subdural hematoma; encephalitis; vascular lesions; cerebral atrophy; trauma to brain with resultant scar tissue forming an epileptogenous focus; depressed skull fracture; foreign bodies; cysts

46. *Observe body for tetany*—a tonic spasm of muscles intermittent, irregular, lasting a few seconds to several hours and days unless relieved. Unilateral, bilateral, generalized, local, or shifting

Integrity of motor, sensory and autonomic nerves

Parathyroid disease; low blood calcium; infections; gastrointestinal conditions; toxemias (ergot, lead, alcohol, morphine, chloroform, uremia) Pregnancy; rickets

47. *Test the following tendon reflexes:* with a percussion hammer: supraorbital, jaw, pectoral, biceps, triceps, radial, ulnar

Klippel-Weil sign. Forcibly extend flexed contractured fingers. In pyramidal lesions, the thumb will flex and adduct

Hoffman sign—pinch and snap nail of index or middle finger. In pyramidal lesions, the terminal phalanx of the thumb is flexed and adducted

Deep tendon reflexes. Integrity of reflex nervous pathways. Chart reflex findings estimating response from O-4 (clonus) by placing right side results as numerator of the fraction and left as denominator

Upper motor neuron diseases; (pyramidal tract—reflexes will be increased) *Lower motor neuron diseases;* (anterior horn cell disease; spinal root; peripheral nerve) reflexes will be reduced or absent). In high strung persons reflexes may be increased

48. At this time, examine heart, lungs, blood pressure

Integrity of heart, lungs, and blood pressure mechanism

Cardiac, pulmonary, and cardiovascular diseases

49. Examine abdomen

Abdominal pathology

Abdominal diseases

50. Abdominal reflex. With patient on his back and relaxed and using a blunt object as a wooden applicator or a toothpick,

Abdominal reflex. Normally the umbilicus deviates to the side stimulated. May be absent in obese, multiparous and

Pyramidal tract lesions produce absent reflex

Spinal cord lesions at level of segment serving reflex

Test	*Testing*	*For*
stroke the skin of the upper, lateral, abdomen outward and downward parallel to the costal arch. In lower abdomen, stroke upward and outward. *Abdominal reflexes:* Abdominal muscles contract toward the side stimulated	elderly patients and those with abdominal scars	
51. Observe and palpate legs with patient on back	Skin condition, color varicosities, symmetry, deformities, joint abnormalities, atrophy, hypertrophy, and abnormal movements. Palpate muscles for tenderness and tone	Variety of conditions
52. Kick my hand with your right leg stiff— now your left. (Hold your hand about 2 ft. above the leg)	Mobility, muscle tone, spasticity, rigidity, muscle strength, coordination and presence or absence of pain	Variety of conditions as spasticities; rigidities; weaknesses; inflammations; bone and joint conditions
53. Raise your leg and shake it	Spasticity, rigidity, weakness, coordination	Same as #52
54. With your eyes open first, then closed, place the heel on the opposite knee and run it down the shin of that leg. Now the other heel	Integrity of posterior columns of spinal cord and cerebellar pathways	*Posterior Column Disease:* Patient can perform test better with eyes open as the eyes compensate for the deficiency in position sense

Cerebellar Disease: No improvement in test performance with eyes open |

55. Bend your toes up, now down (against resistance of examiner's hand) repeat with opposite leg. Bend your knee (with leg held down by examiner's hand). Bend your knee up tight now straighten your leg out (against resistance). Spread your legs apart (against resistance). Now push your legs together (against resistance)	Muscle strength	Any neuromuscular condition causing weakness
56. With lower leg and thigh flexed, extend lower leg on thigh.	Integrity of sciatic nerve meningeal irritation	*Lasègue sign:* Patient will complain of pain, discomfort and resistance in posterior thigh and back if sciatic nerve is irritated *Meningeal irritation:* Pain in back and neck will occur, with resistance *(Kernig's sign)*
57. Place heel on opposite knee and push flexed knee down towards examining table	Integrity of hip joint	Hip joint disease. Patrick Sign
58. With pin, wisp of cotton, and temperature tubes, test each leg—then compare, starting on outer upper side of leg progressively down to sole of foot—then up the inner side of leg.	Superficial sensation	Lesions of peripheral nerves, spinal cord, internal capsule

Test	Testing	For
Genitals and perianal region and buttocks may be tested at this time		
59. Tell me when you don't feel this tuning fork vibrate—place on malleoli, patellae, tibiae and anterior superior iliac spines. Compare the two sides.	Integrity of posterior columns of spinal cord	Subacute combined sclerosis: Multiple sclerosis Tabes dorsalis Spinal cord tumor Rupture of intervertebral disc
60. (With the eyes closed) Do I have one or two fingers on your shin? Measure by cm. right over left	Two point discrimination. Integrity of posterior columns of spinal cord	See #59
61. (With eyes closed) Am I moving your toe up or down?	Position sense. Integrity of posterior columns of spinal cord	See #59
62. Patient recumbent: crook your index finger above the patella and tap the finger with the percussion hammer. If present, patella will be pulled upwards	Deep reflexes. Suprapatelar (normally)	Any lesion that interrupts peripheral pathway to spinal cord and pyramidal tract to cortex
63. Support the under surface of the knees by placing one's arm under the knee to be tested and rest hand on opposite knee— thus mildly flexing the leg to be tested. Then tap the patellar tendon. (With patient sitting on edge of the examining table or chair, tap the tendon)	Deep reflexes. Normally, lower leg extends and quadriceps can be felt to retract	Same as #62

64. Legs are semiflexed and abducted slightly and equally. The examiner places his index finger on the tendons of the semimembranous and semitendinosus muscles. Tap the finger and the leg is flexed and abducted

Deep reflexes. Hamstring

Same as #62

65. Patient recumbent or sitting. Place the Achilles tendon on stretch by placing the hand on the ball of the foot and tapping the tendon

Deep reflexes. Ankle

Same as #62

66. Using a blunt point (applicator, match, dull pin, tooth pick) stroke the sole of the foot upward from the heel. If the defense reaction is too great, flex the leg and place it on the opposite leg. The defense reaction consists of the withdrawal of the foot from the examiner. In some people this is very active as the actual stimulation or even the thought of stimulation of the sole of the foot causes a retraction of the foot. The normal plantar reflex consists of the flexion of the big toe. The plantar reflex

Plantar reflex, Babinski reaction, integrity of pyramidal tract

Same as #62

Test	Testing	For
may not be present in some persons especially those with calloused feet. The Babinski reaction consists of the dorsal extension of the big toe when the sole of the foot is stimulated as noted above—and there is usually a fanning of the toes at the same time		
67. Draw a semicircle around the lower end of the external malleolus with a blunt instrument. Dorsal extension of the big toe occurs when the test is positive	Corroborative tests of the plantar reflex. Chaddock sign	Same as #62
68. With the thumb on the inner surface of the tibia and index finger on the anterior tibial muscles, run these fingers down the leg with firm pressure. Dorsal extension of the big toe will occur when the test is positive	Oppenheim sign	Same as #62
69. Grasp the calf muscles firmly with the thumb and fingers. Dorsal extension of the big toe occurs when the test is positive	The Gordon reflex	Same as #62

| 70. Compress firmly the tendon of Achilles with the fingers. Dorsal extension of the big toe occurs when the test is positive | The Schaefer sign | Same as #62 |
| 71. Examine the back at this point. Have patient sit on edge of table. Note color and texture of skin, posture, vertebral column, etc. Examine back for superficial sensation with pinpoint, wisp of cotton and thermal tubes. Percuss spine with percussion hammer | Integrity and motions of vertebral column, superficial sensation of back, tenderness of spine, muscles, skin, etc. | Any abnormality of vertebral column, sensory system, etc. |

SUMMARY OF NEUROLOGIC EXAMINATION TESTS

1. Stand here, toes and heels together (bare feet). Eyes open then closed.

2. Open eyes. Stand on right foot — now left. Close eyes and repeat.

3. Open eyes. Jump up and down on right foot — now left foot.

4. Walk naturally across room and back again.

5. Walk heel to toe in a straight line across room like this (demonstrate).

6. Walk on toes — now on heels.

7. Walk sidewise to the right lifting your foot up each time — then to the left.

8. Squat down to the floor.

9. Examine head, listen to head with stethoscope, run the fingers over the head and percuss head.

10. Examine scalp with pin.

11. Examine head with a tuning fork. First on the top of the head and over both mastoid processes.

12. Examine the eyes — general appearance, ocular tension test, listen to the eyes with a stethoscope, corneal reflex, extraocular movements, light reflex, fundus examination, test for diplopia, visual fields test, visual acuity test.

13. Wrinkle your forehead up, frown, close your eyes, show your teeth, sniff and move your nostrils in and out, blow your cheeks, purse your lips, whistle, pull your ears back.

14. Examine tongue for taste.

15. Have patient bite hard on both sides of the mouth on a tongue blade and palpate actions of the masseter and temporal muscles on both sides.

16. Test superficial sensation of forehead and face.

17. Examine face for skin color, texture, dryness, wetness, or atrophy of facial tissue.

18. Examine mouth and pharnyx.

19. Note quality of voice.

20. Have patient rotate head to both sides while testing sternocleido-mastoid muscles.

21. Have patient shrug shoulders up and down with and without resistance.

22. Examine tongue, position of protruded tongue, status of muscle, status of muscles of tongue, and range of motion of tongue. Observe tongue for involuntary, abnormal muscular action.

23. Examine neck for any abnormalities.

24. Examine arms with arms extended in front of patient, testing muscular strength of fingers, hands, wrists, elbows, and shoulders.

25. Rotate the forearms back and forth.

26. Finger to nose test.

27. Superficial sensation test of arms.

28. Test for hysterical sensation.

29. Test arms and fingers for deep sensation.

30. Test hands for stereognosis.

31. Examine arms and shoulders for muscle status.

32. Examine shoulders, arms, hands, body and legs for fibrillary twitch-ings, tremors, choreic and athetoid motions, habit and reflex spasms, dystonic motions, and for convulsive motions and tetany.

33. Examine muscles of arms for muscle tone, irritability of muscles and muscle consistency.

34. Examine deep tendon reflexes of arms.

35. Examine heart, lungs, and blood pressure.

36. Examine abdomen.

37. Examine the abdominal reflexes.

38. Observe and palpate legs with patient on the back in a recumbent position.

39. Test the ability of the legs to perform various tests for coordination, muscle strength, range of motion, etc.

40. Perform the heel to knee test with eyes open then closed.

41. Test for muscle strength of the toes, feet, and legs.

42. Examine the legs for Kernig sign, Patrick sign and Laségue sign.

43. Examine superficial sensation of legs.

44. Examine deep sensation of legs.

45. Examine deep tendon reflexes of leg.

46. Examine the Plantar reflex and perform the Babinski test with its modifications.

47. Examine skin, soft tissues of the back, vertebral column, range of motion of the back and for points of tenderness.

4. *Neurologic Diagnostic Reminders and Case Histories*

SINCE THIS WORK is a manual and not a textbook on neurology, the author thought that this chapter might be devoted to a few common neurologic signs, their interpretation and a few case histories representative of neurologic conditions. Since the author has described most of the major neurologic conditions in Chapter 2 in conjunction with an interpretation of the symptoms of the patient and what neurologic conditions are brought to mind, it is not necessary to make a detailed listing of the major neurologic disorders and a description of each. This would only be repetition.

To quote Dr. Israel S. Wechsler, one of my neurologic teachers:

In order to arrive at a direct diagnosis of neurologic condition, a *systematic* examination of the patient is perhaps more important than in any other field of medicine. No other branch lends itself so well to the correlation of signs and symptoms with disease structure, but only through methodical examination can one elicit all of them or properly determine most of them. Certainly in neurology less than in any other specialty may one permit himself a 'snap' diagnosis. It may be conceded that no amount of method ever made a neurologist but it is equally certain that the want of it often marred one. Some persons, fortunately, are endowed with a keen diagnostic sense. (This really consists of a very rapid, almost 'unconscious' logical thinking based on extensive experience.) In general it can only be gained through scientific discipline in repeated practical examination of patients.

Dr. Wechsler, further on in his textbook of clinical neurology, makes the following observations:

Owing to the tremendous growth of neurology as a specialty the fact is sometimes overlooked that it is closely linked with internal medicine. Indeed a neurological diagnosis frequently can only be based upon a sound knowledge of medicine, the neurological condition in many instances being merely the incidental expression of an underlying general pathologic state. To make a diagnosis of hemiplegia and ignore the nephritis or endocarditis which may be the cause of it, or to overlook pernicious anemia in stating that the patient has combined sclerosis, is to show skill in neurological technique without practicing medicine. A more correct point of view is to regard every patient who shows neurological symptoms as a medical 'case.' Therefore every neurological status should include an examination of the heart and lungs, palpation of the pulse and abdomen, search for palpable glands, investigation of the shape and contour of the skull, examination of the urine, blood pressure and temperature determination, sometimes a rectal or vaginal examination, and occasionally a complete blood count or blood chemistry determination or an x-ray examination. Finally, a complete and detailed history is almost as essential as an examination. While it is unwise to jump at conclusions, an accurate history often points to a diagnosis even before a neurological examination has been completed.

Grinker, in his book *Neurology*, makes the following statement:

In general medicine, symptoms and signs of disease processes are for the most part positive in nature. That is, the disease manifests itself by some indication of its presence, inherent in itself. A carcinoma of the stomach produces a palpable mass, pain and bleeding. Typhoid fever is characterized by manifestations of the toxic products of the organisms and the lesions it produces in the intestines. In addition there is, of course, considerable evidence of damage of the organ involved. Neurological diagnosis, however, differs markedly. The disease is not manifested to us by signs of itself, but by its effects on normal function. The pathological process produces destruction within the nervous system. The result of such lesion is the production of signs of lost function, corresponding to the area destroyed, and signs of abnormal activity due to the release of lower structures which have been inhibited by the functional activity of the area destroyed. The lesion produces, then, a negative effect due to destruction and a positive effect due to release.

It is a maxim in neurologic diagnosis that more mistakes are made from not looking and examining than by not knowing. One should always do a complete neurologic examination even if a few symptoms and signs seem to be pathognomonic of one disease.

The author thought it might be helpful to have a short list of neurologic diagnostic reminders as a quick and easy guide to occupational physicians.

Neurologic Signs	*Diagnostic Reminders*
Nystagmus	Multiple sclerosis — congenital nystagmus has been present since birth-cerebral, cerebellar and other posterior fossa tumors, medullary and pontine lesions can also cause nystagmus at times; high cervical cord lesions may produce nystagmus — may be occular, vestibular, cerebral or cerebellar.

Neurologic Signs

Diplopia

Diagnostic Reminders,

Multiple sclerosis — virus infection causing paralysis of the abducens nerve (6th cranial nerve), tumors of the cerebellopontine angle, base of the brain, pons and medulla—fractures at the base of the skull—cerebral hemorrhage—encephalitis—meningitis—thrombosis of the cavernous sinus. Migrainous ophthalmoplegia—syphillis has always been the most common cause and still must be thought of in differential diagnosis.

Pupillary Pathology

AR (Argyll-Robertson) pupil seen in tabes dorsalis and paresis — fixed pupil — meningo-vascular or cerebrospinal syphilis tonic dilated pupil — part of Adie's syndrome in which loss of ankle jerks may also occur.

Unilateral dilation — tumor on the same side, fracture of the skull, hemorrhage of the brain.

Bilateral contraction — tabes dorsalis, cerebral arteriosclerosis, morphine and morphine derivatives.

Unilateral contraction — Horner's syndrome (with enophthalmos).

Reduced Vision

Errors in refraction, optic atrophy, papill edema, optic neuritis, retrobulbar neuritis, retinal and choroidal changes, and hysteria.

Optic Atrophy

Multiple sclerosis, pituitary and parasellar tumors, tabes dorsalis, toxic, occasionally frontal lobe tumors.

Papilledema

Brain tumor, abscess of the brain, encephalitis, cerebral hemorrhage, fracture of the skull, meningitis, inflammation of the optic nerve behind the eyeball.

Retrobulbar Neuritis

Infection, secondary from adjacent foci, usually the sinuses are the chief cause. "The patient sees nothing and the doctor sees nothing" is a good reminder to remember. However, as the neuritis progresses, changes are seen in the disc by the examiner

Optic Neuritis	Inflammation of the optic nerve within the eyeball. Usually caused by syphilis, albuminuria, anemia, leukemia and diabetes. The disc is red and the margins are blurred.
Restriction of the Visual Fields	Transitory and periodic migraine must be considered. If permanent and progressive — brain tumor, brain abscess, subdural hematoma (with a history of previous head injury), multiple sclerosis (enlarged blind spots also occur).
Tender Areas of the Head	Previous head injury — bony pathology of the skull from bone disease, brain tumors, malignancy, etc.
Facial Weakness (Lower 2/3)	Pyramidal tract lesion (cortex to facial nucleus) such as a cerebral vascular lesion-hemorrhage or thrombosis—brain tumor, brain abscess, subdural hematoma.
Facial Weakness (Complete Face)	Bell's palsy—peripheral nerve lesion (facial nucleus to facial musculature.
Rinne Test Positive	Occlusion of the external canal of that external or middle ear.
Weber Test Lateralized (Spontaneously)	Middle ear disease or occlusion of the external canal from some blocking of the conduction system — bone conduction better than air conduction.
Nasal Voice	Cleft palate — some obstruction or condition of the nose or pharynx — brain stem lesion such as vascular, degenerative, neoplastic (anterior horn cell or peripheral nerve) — myasthenia gravis.
Atrophy (One Side of the Tongue)	Progressive muscular atrophy, amyotrophic lateral sclerosis — peripheral nerve lesion with anterior horn cell lesion.
Unequal Tendon Reflexes	*Hyperreflexia* — pyramidal tract pathology from *pressure* of expanding lesions of brain or spinal cord, or rupture of an intervertebral disc; from *degeneration* (multiple sclerosis, amyotrophic lateral sclerosis, subacute combined sclerosis, etc.)

Neurologic Signs	Diagnostic Reminders
Reduced Sensation	Peripheral neuritis, neuropathy, spinal cord disease, cranial nerve disease, brain lesions.
Increased Sensation	Causalgia—herpes zoster—irritative thalamic and other brain lesions—peripheral neuritis—trigeminal neuralgia—trigger areas on face from trigeminal neuralgia.
Reduced Muscle Strength	Brain tumors—abscesses—vascular lesions—degenerations and injuries—peripheral neuritis—peripheral nerve injuries—inflammation or degenerations of anterior horn cells—myositis.
Increased Muscle Tone	Pyramidal tract lesions; Parkinsonism.
Muscle Atrophy	Atrophy from disuse as in sciatic neuritis or hip pathology — amyotrophic lateral sclerosis, progressive muscular atrophy (chronic polio), peripheral nerve injury.
Fibrillary Twitchings	Amyotrophic lateral sclerosis — progressive muscular atrophy, pressure from a ruptured intervertebral disc.
Unsteady Gait	Tabes dorsalis—multiple sclerosis, subacute combined degeneration, cerebellar disease (tumor or degeneration).
Dragging Feet	Peroneal palsy (dropped foot), pyramidal tract lesion due to tumor, degeneration, vascular or injury, peripheral neuritis or neuropathy.
Babinski Toe Reflex	Pyramidal tract lesion.
Intention Tremor	Multiple sclerosis.
Rest Tremor (Pill Rolling)	Parkinsonism.
Inability to Adduct Little Finger	Ulnar nerve palsy.
Inability to Flex Distal Phalanx of Index Finger	Median nerve palsy.
Inability to Dorsiflex Hand at Wrist	Radial nerve palsy.
Inability to Dorsiflex Foot and Toes (Foot Drop)	Common peroneal nerve palsy.

Inability to Plantarflex Foot and Toes	Tibial nerve palsy.
Mask Facies	Parkinsonism
Decreased Associated Motions of Arms While Walking	Parkinsonism
Rigid Body While Walking	Parkinsonism
One Arm, Flexed at Elbow Held Close to Body	Cerebral vascular disease, brain tumor and other conditions involving pyramidal tract.
Facial Ties (Involuntary Twitchings of Facial Muscles)	Psychogenic origin, emotional instability.
Fainting	Because fainting occurs often enough in occupational medicine, the author thought that a more detailed discussion of the differential diagnosis of syncope was in order.

FAINTING

Fainting occurs often enough amongst employees at the work place to warrant a brief discussion. For the purposes of this manual I have taken some thoughts expressed by Engel in his classic monograph titled *Fainting*.* He defines fainting as follows, "Hence in this monograph all the conditions in which symptoms as giddiness, lightheadedness, and related symptoms occur, as well as the conditions characterized regularly by complete loss of consciousness and falling will be considered as examples of syncope."

Engel continues, "Syncope is only a symptom and may be due to a wide variety of causes. Most often it represents only one manifestation of an underlying pathologic process. The most convenient classification of syncope is based on mechanisms rather than on etiology. Three basic mechanisms account for all examples. These are:

1. Altered cerebral metabolism due to circulatory disturbances.
2. Altered cerebral metabolism due to metabolic factors.
3. Psychologic mechanisms not involving any known disturbance in cerebral metabolism or circulation.

For clinical purposes, Engel mentioned the following types of syncope.

1. Fall in arterial blood pressure.
2. Cardiac standstill.
3. Cerebral vascular disorders.
4. Cerebral metabolic disorders.
5. Hysteria.

*Engel, G. L.: Fainting — Physiological and Psychological Considerations, ed. 2. *Publisher*, Springfield, Ill., Charles C Thomas.

6. Hyperventilation.
7. Heart disease (excluding Adams-Stokes syndrome).
A few facts about each of these types are as follows:

1. Fall in Arterial Blood Pressure.

Three sub-types are recognized:
1. Vasodepressor syncope, the most common type of fainting, occurs in settings experienced as danger, when escape or activity is impossible or when fear must be denied; usually occurs in response to fear, anxiety, pain, injury, sight of blood, viewing accidents etc.; symptoms usually occur in the erect position and consist of muscular weakness epigastric discomfort, nausea, sweating, restlessness, sighing respiration, yawning, lightheadedness, blurring of vision, loss of consciousness and convulsions if unconsciousness is prolonged; treatment is usually not necessary since spontaneous recovery is usually rapid, but if recovery is delayed patient should be examined for injury, tissue damage, loss. of blood or vasodilatation.
2. Orthostatic hypotension is characterized by chronic or repetitive fainting upon assuming the upright position due to inadequate compensatory mechanisms to maintain circulation to the head — such conditions as inadequate postural reflex, chronic anxiety states, prolonged recumbency and convalescence, pregnancy in the first trimester, etc.
3. Increase in intrathoracic pressure, a rare cause of spontaneous syncope, is caused by a paroxysm of coughing amongst children with pertussis and adults with chronic laryngitis or bronchitis. Work which entails blowing against pressure might also be a cause of this type of syncope.

2. Cardiac Standstill

1. Adams-Stoke syndrome.
2. Reflex heart block occurs from hypersensitivity or stimulation of any portion of the reflex arc synapsing with the vagus nucleus such as cardioinhibitory carotid sinus syncope, vagovagal syncope, oculovagal syncope, etc.

3. Cerebral vascular disorders

These disorders result from a transient cerebral vasospasm or reduced blood flow; neurologic signs and symptoms may occur; types may be the cerebral type of carotid sinus reflex hypersensitivity, migraine, hypertension, cerebral vascular disease, brain tumors, carotid and/or vertebral artery thrombosis.

4. Disturbances in cerebral metabolism

Dizziness, lightheadedness or faintness is common, but unconsciousness is not; types are anoxemia, chronic anemia, hypoglycemia, delirium.

5. Hysterical fainting

More common among women, and unintelligent and culturally unsophisticated people; other characteristics of hysterical character structure are often present. This type of syncope may be contagious in settings where many people work.

6. Hyperventilation

Hyperventilation is often psychogenic in origin, but may occur in essentially healthy individuals or in hysterical persons as a general physiological reaction to fear, anger or pain; it may occur in a response to certain drugs such as salicylate in delirious patients.

7. *Heart disease*

Most patients who faint do not have heart disease. However, since heart disease is the most frequent cause of sudden death perhaps it would be more accurate to say that fainting with heart disease actually is common but the first attack is usually fatal; fainting with heart disease must therefore be regarded as an ominous sign; the coexistence of fainting in a cardiac lesion does not necessarily relate the two; anxiety in the cardiac patient may lead either to vasodepressor syncope or to hyperventilation.

Engel also devotes a small chapter to fainting during air travel. He states that in both civilian and military flight fainting is an occasional occurrence and that it is well for the physician to be familiar with the different types of syncope and the various factors responsible. He mentions the following types of syncope— anxiety, anoxia, abdominal distention, Eustachian tube and sinus blockage, decompression sickness and centrifugal force.

Briefly, in summary one might say:

1. The most common type of syncope is vasodepressor.
2. Only a small proportion of patients with vasodepressor syncope actually lose consciousness.
3. When the patient complains of having fainted but once or twice the diagnostic possibilities are broad.
4. In repetitive fainting, however, only a few types account for most cases, such as, neurotic, either vasodepressor, hysterical or hyperventilation.
5. Neurotic fainting usually begins early in life around puberty and rarely after 35 years of age.
6. Neurotic fainting beginning after 35 years of age is rare.
7. When repeated fainting begins after middle life, organic disease of the heart, cerebral blood vessels and vagus and sympathetic reflex pathways are the most likely causes.
8. Among men vasodepressor syncope is more common, while among women hysterical syncope and hyperventilation are more common.

Engel lists the following conditions in differential diagnosis, namely, epilepsy vertigo, narcolepsy, cataplexy, familial periodic paralysis and schizophrenia.

Once again, the author wishes to express his acknowledgement of the fact that the material in this section was taken from Engel's monograph on Fainting. If more information is desired on this subject, the monograph is highly recommended.

NEUROLOGIC CASE HISTORIES

The following brief neurologic case histories are presented at this time to represent the more common neurologic conditions seen at the work place.

MULTIPLE SCLEROSIS

1. *Male, 37, married, 2 young children*
   1. Poor balance and walking difficulty, 1st symptom, 9 years ago.
   2. Diplopia, 3rd year of illness.
   3. Numbness of left fingers, 4th year.
   4. Speech became slurred and thick, 6th year.
   5. Numbness of right hand, 8th year.
   6. Inability to walk and to use hands, in a wheel chair, 9th year.
   7. Nicotinamide, 50 mg. q.i.d., produced generalized flushing, patient felt better.
   8. Placed on total and permanent disability.

2. *Female, 23, single*
   1. Numbness of hands, 1st symptom, 6 years ago.
   2. Numbness of whole body, next symptom.
   3. A "band" feeling around waist.
   4. Diplopia.
   5. Legs and arms became weak and stiff.
   6. Difficulty walking and writing, 3rd year.
   7. Unsteady, spastic gait, 3rd year.
   8. Above symptoms fluctuated widely.
   9. Married, 4th year of disease.
   10. Delivered full term baby, 5th year of disease.
   11. Symptoms remained as above.
   12. Nicotinamide, 50 mg. t.i.d., helped patient feel better.
   13. Patient worked until she left for pregnancy, remained at home.

3. *Male, 26, single*
   1. Numbness and tingling of lower legs and feet, first symptom, 8 years ago.
   2. Numbness of thighs, 2nd symptom, 1 month later.
   3. Two point perception poor on legs, first year.
   4. Numbness fluctuated first year.
   5. Visual blurring, 2nd year.
   6. Numbness, right face, 2nd year.
   7. Numbness, left face, 3rd year.
   8. Diplopia, 5th year.
   9. Dizziness, 5th year.
   10. Blind spot developed in left eye, 5th year.
   11. Left arm weak and stiff, 6th year.
   12. Balance poor, standing and walking, 6th year.
   13. Field of vision restricted, right, 6th year.

14. Unsteady gait, 6th year.
15. All above symptoms fluctuate.
16. Patient still working, employer knows of condition.
17. Patient married, 5th year of disease.

4. *Male, 28, married, one child*
 1. Blindness, left eye, intermittent, 1st symptom, 1 year ago.
 2. Numbness, right fingers, intermittent, 1st year.
 3. Numbness, left fingers, intermittent, 2nd year.
 4. Working regularly.
 5. Nicotinamide, 50 mg., q.i.d., helped patient.
 6. Patient working, employer knows of condition.

5. *Male, 28, married, 2 young children*
 1. Retrobulbar neuritis, bilateral, diagnosed at first, 2 years ago.
 2. Diplopia, intermittent, 3rd year.
 3. Buzzing, left ear, intermittent, 3rd year.
 4. Poor balance, 4th year.
 5. Numbness, right foot, 4th year.
 6. Scotoma developed in right visual field, 4th year.
 7. Poor vision, right eye, 4th year.
 8. Poor walking, stiff and weak legs, 5th year.
 9. Incoordination, in a wheel chair, 6th year.
 10. Nicotinamide, no help.
 11. Placed on total and permanent disability.

CONVULSIVE DISORDER

6. *Male, 26, married*
 1. First convulsion at 10 years of age, grand mal type.
 2. Last convulsion, 13 months before office visit.
 3. Neurologic examination negative.
 4. Electroencephalogram (EEG) negative.
 5. Working regularly, employer knows of condition.
 6. Convulsions controlled by phenobarbital, gr. ½ t.i.d.

7. *Male, 50, married, 3 children*
 1. Nocturnal convulsions, grand mal, for 27 years.
 2. No daytime convulsions.
 3. Neurologic exam negative.
 4. EEG positive for convulsive disorder.
 5. Convulsions controlled by Dilantin, Sodium, gr. 4½ at bedtime.
 6. Over fatigue or excessive worry may produce a nocturnal convulsion.
 7. Working regularly and employer knows of condition.

8. *Female, 40, single*

1. Grand mal and petit mal convulsions for 25 years.
2. Convulsions precipitated by worry.
3. Neurologic exam negative.
4. EEG, positive, for convulsive disorder.
5. Controlled by Dilantin, Sodium, gr. 1½ t.i.d. and Phenobarbital, gr. ½ t.i.d.
6. Working regularly and employer knows of condition.

PARKINSONISM (PARALYSIS AGITANS)

9. *Male, 35, single*

1. Constant, rhythmic tremor, left arm, hand, fingers, leg (hemi-Parkinsonism) 10 years.
2. Attacks of "eyes being pulled up and out and stuck there" for 1-5 minutes (oculogyric crisis).
3. Mask facies, for years.
4. Drooling of mouth, occasionally, for 10 years.
5. Rabellon helped the tremor and rigidities.
6. Benzedrine helped the eye attacks.
7. Patient still working and employer knows of condition.

10. *Female, 62, married*

1. Weakness and rigidity of arms and legs, gradual development, 2 years.
2. On arising, takes 2-3 steps backwards (retropulsion). While walking forward, she is so rigid that she walks too fast and has to grab something to prevent falling (anteropulsion).
3. Stares straight ahead.
4. Mask facies, no facial expressions at all.
5. Slight "pill rolling" tremor, left hand and fingers.
6. Skin of hands and fingers, smooth and glistening.
7. Worked regularly till 6 months ago.

PERIPHERAL NEUROPATHY

11. *Female, 38, married*

1. Tingling, 4th and 5th fingers, ulnar ½ of right hand and forearm, 3 months.
2. Hypalgesia, ulnar area, right hand and forearm.
3. Atrophy, interossei, right greater than left.
4. Pain, both shoulders, right greater than left.
5. Lost 45 lbs. weight in 1½ years.
6. Axillary glands enlarged.

7. Hodgkins Disease diagnosed and treated in hospital.

8. *Diagnosis:* Radiculitis, cervical 7th and 8th roots and thoracic first root.

12. *Female, 35, married, 2 children*

1. Pins and needles, right arm, 2 weeks.
2. Weakness and heaviness, right arm, 1 week.
3. Pain, right arm, 1 week.
4. Aching, right shoulder, neck, upper back, 1 week.
5. Headache, dizziness, 1 week.
6. Tender areas, right shoulder, neck.
7. *Diagnosis:* Brachial plexus neuritis.

13. *Male, 53, married*

1. Numbness, tingling, 4th and 5th fingers, both hands and ulnar area of forearm, 4 weeks.
2. Weakness, mild, 4th and 5th fingers, bilaterally, 4 weeks.
3. Hypalgesia, both ulnar areas.
4. Atrophy, mild, interossei.
5. *Diagnosis:* Pressure neuropathy (chronic, pressure on both ulnar nerves in elbow area) patient was an inveterate chess player and leaned on both elbows extensively while playing chess.

14. *Female, 55, married*

1. Numbness, 4th and 5th fingers, right hand, 4 weeks.
2. Weakness, decreased use, right arm, 3 weeks.
3. Can't pick things up or lift with right hand, 3 weeks.
4. Pain, tenderness, right shoulder, neck and arm, 3 weeks.
5. Patchy areas of reduced sensation, right arm.
6. Reflexes reduced, right arm.
7. *Diagnosis:* Brachial neuritis, acute, right.

15. *Male, 42, married, 3 children*

1. Pain in lower back, right leg (posterior) acute, following lifting, 3 days.
2. Weakness, right leg and painful walking.
3. Tenderness, lower right back, and back of right leg.
4. Reduced ankle jerk.
5. Reduced superficial sensation (pin, cotton, thermal) posterior, right thigh.
6. *Diagnosis:* (1) Sciatic neuritis, acute, right, secondary to (2) ruptured intervertebral disc.

16. *Male, 54, married, 4 children*
   1. Pain, right, posterior leg acute and "achy" at times, 3 weeks.
   2. Can't sit long as leg hurts.
   3. Tender areas in right lower back, buttock, posterior right leg.
   4. Reduced ankle jerk and superficial sensation.
   5. Rest, heat and analgesics helped patient.
   6. *Diagnosis:* Sciatic neuritis, right, acute.

POST-TRAUMATIC ENCEPHALOPATHY (HEAD SYNDROME, CONCUSSION SYNDROME)

17. *Female, 24, single*
   1. Head caught in a subway door, unconscious for a few minutes.
   2. Headaches, dizziness, weakness, insomnia, nightmares of subway doors clanging and banging, changes in posture develop dizziness and headache.
   3. Irritable, tense and anxious.
   4. Neurologic exam negative.
   5. X-ray skull negative.
   6. Gradually improved and returned to work.

18. *Male, 40, married, one child*
   1. While driving auto, patient's ear was hit on left side.
   2. Head and entire left side of body injured.
   3. In a "daze" for 1 hour following accident.
   4. Headaches, dizziness, increased irritability, fatiguability, weakness for a few weeks.
   5. Gradually improved.

CEREBRAL NEOPLASM

19. *Male, 60, married*
   1. Twitching, right face, 3 months.
   2. Difficulty in saying what he wants to say, 3 weeks.
   3. Progressive weakness, right side of body, 3 weeks.
   4. Vomiting, with no nausea, or stomach disorder, 3 weeks.
   5. Motor aphasia, right spastic hemiparesis.
   6. Headache, progressively worse.
   7. *Diagnosis:* Metastatic carcinoma, left fronto-parieto-temporal, from bronchogonic carcinoma, left lung.

20. *Female, 42, single*
   1. Headaches, blurred vision, 4 weeks.
   2. Weakness, left arm, 2 weeks.
   3. Weakness, left leg, 1 week.
   4. X-ray skull showed pineal gland calcified and shifted to left of midline.

5. Left hemipareis with increased reflexes.

6. *Diagnosis:* Cerebral tumor, spongioblastoma, right cerebrum infiltrating.

FACIAL NEURALGIA

21. *Male, 45 married*

1. Pains, lightning like, sharp, sudden, left face, 2 months.

2. Pain starts between left eye and ear, then travels between eye and ear, into neck, face and head, 2 months.

3. Pain triggered by chewing and occasionally by a gust of wind.

4. Pain lasts from 3-24 hours, average is 10 hours.

5. Tender face, ache in left ear during attacks.

6. Neurologic exam negative.

7. Trigeminal nerve sectioned with complete relief.

22. *Female, 61, married*

1. Pain, severe, attacks in right face, lower third, sudden onset.

2. Triggered by rubbing face.

3. Pain lasts 1-6 hours, relieved by nothing.

4. Trigeminal nerve sectioned, pain relieved, but patient complains of right face being "woodeny and burning."

SPASMODIC TORTICOLLIS

23. *Male, 50, married*

1. Spasmodic, irregular pulling of head and chin to left, 6 months.

2. Highly tense person, emotionally unstable, immature.

3. Divorced, remarried.

4. Job difficulties.

5. Psychotherapy and tranquilizers helped.

6. Working regularly.

MIGRAINE

24. *Male, 32, married, 4 children*

1. Attacks of blinding scotomata, followed by severe left sided headache, nausea, vomiting.

2. Father had migraine.

3. Patient, highly tense, restless, conscientious, ambitious.

4. Worry over many on-the-job and off-the-job problems.

5. Helped with psychotherapy.

25. *Male, 38, married*

1. Migraine attacks, 20 years, every 1-2 weeks.

2. Tense, emotional and worrisome of life's problems.

3. Depressive tendency and 2 prolonged hospitalizations for depressions.
4. Helped with psychotherapy.

AMYOTROPHIC LATERAL SCLEROSIS

26. *Male, 62, married, 2 children*
    1. Weakness, left ankle, dragged left foot, 1st symptom, 4 years ago.
    2. Weakness, left leg with increasing stiffness, 1st year.
    3. Later, weakness, stiffness, right leg, 1st year.
    4. Walking difficulty, progressively worse, 1st year.
    5. Fibrillary twitchings, legs, 2nd year.
    6. Weakness, stiffness, arms, 2nd year.
    7. Fibrillary twitchings, arms, 3rd year.
    8. Worked 3 years, then impossible.
    9. Placed on permanent and total disability.

CEREBRAL HEMORRHAGE

27. *Female, 52, widow, one child*
    1. Weak left arm, left leg recovered almost completely.
    2. Stiff left arm.
    3. Walks fairly well with left leg, dragging left foot slightly.
    4. Back on job in office doing everything but typing.
    5. Speech has recovered.

28. *Male, 60, married*
    1. Right spastic hemiparesis, following cerebral hemorrhage.
    2. Speech disturbances.
    3. Had had hypertension for years.
    4. Unemployable now.

MERALGIA PARESTHETICA

29. *Male, 56, married*
    1. Numbness and burning, left thigh, 2 years.
    2. Numbness and burning, right thigh, 2 months.
    3. Neurologic exam negative.
    4. May be due to obesity, pressure on lateral femoral cutaneous nerve.
    5. Usually, patients learn to live with this symptom.

BELL'S PALSY

30. *Male, 40, single*
    1. While shaving in morning, notices right face paralyzed.
    2. Thought he had a stroke, became tense and excited.
    3. Right face "numb" and completely paralyzed, including forehead.
    4. Right eye could hardly be closed, was watering.
    5. Reassured, treated and recovered.

5. *Neurologic Treatment Reminders*

NEUROLOGIC TREATMENT at the workplace, whether this is industry, colleges, governmental agencies, department stores, banks, union, etc., will, for the most part, be very limited. In most instances, the medical department functions as a health maintenance department, and the employee with a neurologic diagnosis or a suspected neurologic diagnosis will be referred to the community neurologist or the family physician. Medical departments in industry or in other places of work are content today to make the diagnosis and then to refer the employee for treatment in the community. However, there are a few companies where the medical department performs complete medical care for employees and occasionally for the dependents also. In companies which are in isolated areas of the country, this type of industrial medical practice may be a necessity. Nevertheless, there are many instances where it would be to the employee's benefit to have limited treatment carried on inside the plant providing this meets with the approval of the family physician or the neurologist. The facilities of the community may be inadequate to treat the employee adequately or the employee would lose too much time from his work if he took treatment outside the plant.

Physical therapy measures and intramuscular injections of various medications constitute the bulk of the therapy. A list of neurologic disorders that might be treated within the plant under certain circumstances might read as follows:

DISEASE	TREATMENT AT WORK
1. *Bell's palsy*	Infrared to the face — or short wave diathermy to the face
	Massage, to the face
	Teaching of facial muscle exercises before the mirror
	Galvanic motor point stimulation of the face (when equipment is available)
	Intramuscular injections of vitamin B_1 or B_{12}
	Psychotherapy
	Mild tranquilizer

DISEASE	TREATMENT AT WORK
2. *Painful Neck and Shoulder Syndromes* due to spasms of muscles from emotional tension.	Short wave diathermy to the neck and shoulder or Infrared Massage of neck and shoulder muscles Neck traction Psychotherapy
3. *Brachial Neuritis*	Infrared or Short wave diathermy Massage to affected muscles Intramuscular injections of vitamin B_1 and/or B_{12} Mild tranquilizer Analgesics for managing pain
4. *Neuritis, Neuropathy, and Nerve Injuries:* radial, ulnar, median, sciatic, peroneal, anterior tibial, post-tibial. Post-traumatic or toxic.	Whirlpool bath for affected limb Short wave diathermy Exercises for strengthening affected muscles Intramuscular injections of vitamin B_1 and/or B_{12} Splinting of fingers or wrist if necessary Analgesics for managing pain Mild tranquilizer
5. *Painful Back Conditions:* ruptured intervertebral disc, weak back condition, muscular spasms, sacroiliac conditions, lumbosacral conditions, arthritis causing root pains.	Physiotherapy Psychotherapy
6. *Hemiplegia:* When hemiplegic patients are working at special jobs.	Infrared to arm or leg Short wave diathermy to affected part Exercises for affected parts Psychotherapy
7. *Multiple Sclerosis*	General management including psychotherapy and interpretation of disease to patient and relatives Nicotinamide — to provide generalized flushing, 50 mg. tablets, 1-3

DISEASE	TREATMENT AT WORK

DISEASE

TREATMENT AT WORK

times a day. Patients feel better after daily flushings though they know that this is no cure for the disease

8. *Epilepsy*

General management education and interpretation of condition
  Specific management
  Job placement
  Job follow-up with medical department and industrial relations department
  Anticonvulsant therapy
  Be specific with treatment
  Suggested medicines
For Grand Mal seizures
  1. Dilantin Sodium—usual starting dose gr. 1½ three times a day with meals
  2. Phenobarbital—usual starting dose gr. ½ with meals
Petit Mal seizures
  1. Tridione—usual starting dose gr. 5 with meals
Other anticonvulsive drugs may be tried such as Mebaral, Mesantoin and Mysoline. A complete blood count should be done every six months when patients are on the above anticonvulsive drugs, especially Sodium Dilantin and Tridione. Toxic side effects of Tridione may consist of unusual sensitivity to light, skin rashes, kidney complications, etc. Blood dyscrasias may follow Sodium Dilantin occasionally.

9. *Head Injuries*

General management
  Psychotherapy
  Interpretation of condition
  Job placement and follow-up on job with medical department and industrial relations department

DISEASE

TREATMENT AT WORK

Medicinal therapy
    Daprisal, edrisal, have proved effective in controlling headache, raising spirits, etc.
    Mild tranquilizer

10. *Retrobulbar and Optic Neuritis* following the acute phase whenever patient returns to work.

Oral medication for general support
    Analgesics
    Blood building agents
Intramuscular injections of vitamin B_1 and/or B_{12}
Psychotherapy

11. *Amyotrophic Lateral Sclerosis:* These patients can and do work for some time following the onset of their symptoms, if their motivation and emotional stability are healthy.

Physical therapy for spastic legs
    Whirlpool bath
    Massage
    Short wave diathermy
    Infrared
    Exercises
    General supportive medicinal therapy
    Job transfer to more suitable work if necessary
    Psychotherapy

12. *Subacute Combined Degeneration* (posterior lateral sclerosis)

    Medicinal therapy
    Blood building agents—liver, etc.
    Tranquilizers if necessary
    Physical therapy
    Whirlpool bath for spastic legs
    Short wave diathermy
    Infrared
    Massage
    Exercise
    Psychotherapy
    Job transfer if necessary for suitable work

13. *Trigeminal Neuralgia* (preoperation for root section) (postoperation for root section) facial sensations of drawing, pulling, numbness, tingling, boring and pain.

    Medicinal therapy for attack
    Oral and hypodermic
    Refer to competent neurosurgeon
    Medicinal therapy
        Mild tranquilizer
        Hypnotic

DISEASE	TREATMENT AT WORK
	Analgesics—at times combined with a stimulant is helpful — as dapraisal or edrisal
	Vitamin B$_1$ and/or B$_{12}$ if indicated
	Physical therapy
	Infrared
	Short wave diathermy
	Massage
	Deep x-ray — at times has helped
	Psychotherapy — a big dose
14. *Progressive Muscular Dystrophy:* These patients can and do work productively for years if they want to. Their motivation to work is usually very high.	*Psychotherapy*
	Medical therapy
	Supportive and symptomatic
	Job transfer if necessary for suitable work as disease progresses
15. *Meralgia Paresthetica*	*Medical therapy*
	Analgesics
	Vitamins B$_1$ or B$_{12}$
	Physical therapy
	Infrared
	Short wave diathermy
	Massage
16. *Herpes Zoster* (shingles)	*Analgesic medicine*
	Infrared and possibly diathermy
	A protective covering for the hyperalgesic zone.
	Tranquilizers
	Intravenous administration of 250 cc. of saline which contains 1.9 mg. of histamine acid phosphate which is given in 1½ hours has also helped
17. *Spasmodic Torticollis* (wry neck)	Nicotinic acid and thiamine has also helped
	Tranquilizers
	Psychotherapy
	Diathermy followed by massage of the muscles of the neck, shoulder
	Neck traction with a Sayre traction outfit

6. *Optimum Time Off for Neurologic Disabilities*

THE REMARKS which I shall make on this topic were part of a presentation entitled. "Optimum Time Off from Work for Neurologic and Psychiatric Disabilities," which I prepared for delivery before the American Academy of Occupational Medicine in Washington in 1956. The entire presentation was published in *Industrial Medicine and Surgery*, September 1956, volume 25, Number 9, pp. 408-412.

If we can arrive at some agreement as to optimum time off for certain disabilities, we physicians in industry and other occupations shall have some guide to go by in dealing with each individual case. Also, our anxieties will not be as great nor our frustrations either, when the supervisor, the foreman, the superintendent or the industrial relations department query us as to when John Jones or Mary Smith will be able to return to work.

In the field of neurology and psychiatry, I know of no attempts to classify these conditions in the same fashion as the cardiologists have classified cardiac lesions. This cardiac classification gives the cardiologist and the industrial physician much information as to the present cardiac condition, as to what the future holds for the patient, as to an average expected time for reemployability, and it also gives these physicians some comfort and security. In the neurologic field, we can approximate in many conditions the expected time for improvement or recovever, in the psychiatric field there are so many variables present in the various individual personality structures, in environmental stresses and strains, in a person's reaction to these stresses and strains based on his past and present behavioral experiences, that it is extremely difficult to prognosticate the optimum time for reemployment. In various medical conditions, surgical diseases and orthopedic disorders the expected time of healing of tissues is fairly well known. However, even in these conditions the personality of the patient with the disease, his motivations for or against recovery militate for or against getting well in the usual time and returning to work. Speaking of individual personality structure, this factor must always be kept in mind, as you know, in dealing with any illness. In psychiatric patients, the personality of the individual before his psychiatric illness is very important and must be considered seriously in the diagnosis and prognosis of the condition and in estimating an expected date for his return to work.

What is the policy of your company towards keeping neurologic and psychiatric patients at work and returning them to work after their illness? What is the attitude of your union toward neurologic and psychiatric disorders? What these two groups think about the N.P. patient has a direct bearing on our topic. If either one or both has an enlightened concern for its employees, then ways will be found to bring them back to work on jobs that they can perform. Today, more and more of us in business are learning the wisdom of considering our people as whole men and women and not just "hands." Do you hire hands, or do you hire the whole man? Fear and distrust of neurologic and psychiatric patients on the job is gradually being reduced because experience has shown from actual performances on the job that many of these patients can continue to work while being treated and can return to work and do a creditable job. However, I am realistic enough to realize that there is much education to be done. This is your job and my job. Whenever and wherever we believe that a recovered or a recovering employee with a neurologic or/and psychiatric disability would benefit psychologically and physically from being on the job and the company also would benefit without disrupting production or the department, we should so state. Resistances will be met, and here is where our job of education begins. There are industrial physicians who will not agree with you and me. There will be, as you know, community physicians who will recommend a long time away from the job, preferably in Florida, Bermuda, or California, but you and I know that work is often good medicine, and that the discipline of our normal routine, including our daily job, may be a most important sustaining factor. "Idleness is the devil's workshop." By returning the neurologic or/and psychiatric patient to work as soon as possible, we shall be helping the patient to regain his confidence in himself or herself, and we shall be augmenting the spirital take-home pay as well as the financial take-home pay.

The approach to this problem is a team approach composed of the medical department or/and the community physician, the personnel department, and the supervisor. This team should strive to work together so that the climate of the department to which the employee is return ing, is a warm, sympathetic and understanding one. Each case must be individualized and considered separately.

It is impossible to consider in this monograph all of the neurologic and psychiatric disorders which all of us see in our every day industrial practice. Therefore, I shall discuss only a few of the more prevalent disturbances in my experiences, leaving out many of which some of you may be concerned with at present. I know that in this brief presentation I have left out much information that you may be wondering about.

The neurologic disorders which I shall deal with are as follows:

1. Multiple sclerosis
2. The convulsive disorders
3. Cerebrovascular lesions
4. The peripheral neuritides
5. Cephalalgias
6. Post-traumatic encephalopathy

MULTIPLE SCLEROSIS

Although we may discuss today and in the future some general principles regarding optimum time off for neurologic and psychiatric illnesses, we must constantly bear in mind that each case must be individualized. The will to work for one person may not be as great as that of another. We must recognize this and if possible, try to find out the reasons for poor motivation and correct them. In discussing multiple sclerosis, the principle of individualization certainly plays an important part. In my experience, the will to work in applicants with multiple sclerosis and in employees who develop multiple sclerosis is quite strong. Among employees who develop multiple sclerosis the guiding indices to me for a decision relative to continuing to work are namely; (1) the neurologic systems involved; (2) degree of involvement of these systems; (3) the job and residual skills available; (4) the personality and motivation of the patient; (5) attitude of supervisor. If the symptoms consist of moderate, intermittent, or continuous dysesthesia, of numbness and tingling of one or more extremities, or a mild weakness of an extremity, the employee may be able to continue to work. If these dysesthesiae are severe or the job is such that the finer sensibilities of touch, two point position sense are necessary, then the employee cannot do that job. However, he may be able to do another job for the time being, if one can be found and if supervision is concerned about him.

If diplopia, decreased vision or/and the symptoms of pyramidal tract disturbance, such as weakness and spasticity are present, the employee may not be able to continue to work. Certainly in my experience, if the cerebellar pathways are involved or the sphincters, he will not be able to work. Time off from work may vary then from no time off to permanent and total disability. This, of course, will depend on severity of attack, diffuseness of symptoms, age of first attack and number of previous attacks. The emotional attitude of the multiple sclerosis patient is usually very optimistic, as you know, and they will want to continue to work. Our job then is to protect the patient if his over-enthusiasm is too great without due regard for his health or for the job. His production may suffer. And, we should also protect the supervisor, the management and the co-worker from the overzealous but inefficient worker. The mild case should be out of work from a period of a few days to maybe 3 to 6 weeks. The moderate case may be out from 4 to 8 weeks. The severe case may be out from 8 weeks to an indefinite time. In my experience, most of the employees with multiple sclerosis that I have seen from many companies have been out of work a very short time or have been able to remain on the job.

THE CONVULSIVE DISORDERS

When an employee develops a grand mal, a petit mal or a psychomotor seizure at work, he should be out of work just long enough to have a complete neurologic and psychiatric examination including a brain wave, x-ray of the skull, blood sugar curve, possibly a spinal puncture and any other laboratory examinations that may be indicated. This should take about 2 to 4 weeks. While he is having these examinations, supervision, the personnel department and the medical department should survey the job situation with the view of finding a suitable job for him on his return. Education of supervision and of the co-workers may be necessary to reduce anxiety surrounding the person with a convulsive disorder. In the field of the convulsive disorders, there has always been much fear, apprehension, anxiety and stigmata. The Committee on Industrial Psychiatry of the Group for the Advancement of Psychiatry of which I am a member, has published a report on the person with convulsive seizures at work. I have discussed this point more thoroughly in Chapter 7. This is an attempt to guide personnel people as to this problem in industry. The family physician may wish the employee to remain out of work longer than four weeks. Discrete and tactful handling of this situation then is called for. The employee from all viewpoints, but especially psychologic, should return to work as soon as possible so that he will regain confidence in himself and become a dignified member of society once again.

CEREBROVASCULAR LESIONS

I consider here cerebral hemorrhage, cerebral thrombosis, cerebral spasm and rupture of a cerebral aneurysm. Having survived the initial vascular assault, the employee with mild symptoms and signs, such as transitory motor and sensory changes, mild to no speech disturbances, mild to no personality changes, may be able to return to work in 4 to 8 weeks. Others may be out from 8 weeks to many months, and some never return. Executives, whose decisions have far-reaching implications affecting many people, may be unable to continue to work because of subtle changes such as poor concentration, episodes of irritability, defects of judgement and personality changes. New jobs may have to be found for these handicapped people, but my experience is that they are grateful and efficient workers.

THE PERIPHERAL NEURITIDES

I shall mention only brachial, ulnar and sciatic neuritis. Brachial neuritis is a long, drawn-out condition which disables the patient for many weeks with pain, restriction of motion and insomnia. Some stoical patients may take no time off. Others may take 1 to 2 weeks for the acute attack to subside. If the dominant arm is involved, his usual work may be more difficult to perform. Other work may have to be found temporarily. However, most of these patients should return to work within 2 to 4 weeks.

Ulnar neuritis usually does not keep a man out of work but he may have to have a different job for 4 to 6 weeks until the symptoms recede. Muscular movements served by the ulnar nerve way be impossible to perform so that his usual job may be impossible for him to do. The numbness and tingling usually are not so discomforting that patients can not stay on the job.

Sciatic neuritis may keep an employee from work for 2 to 8 weeks. Mild attacks may cause discomfort but no time off. The type of work also may determine length of time off Recurrent sciatic neuritis from lumbar disc pathology may cause an absence of several weeks for many episodes. If the personality of the sciatic patient is a relatively sound one, he may take only 1 to 2 weeks off. A different kind of a job for the recovering patient with sciatic neuritis in many instances will aid his recovery and will also benefit him psychologically.

CEPHALALGIAS

Migraine and tension headaches are considered. Severe migraine attacks occasionally may keep a person from work for a few days. However, with psychotherapy and occasional help from Gynergen Wygraine and allied medicines, these people can usually be kept at work. Attempts certainly should be made to uncover the emotional causes for the migraine attacks. Severe tension headaches, however, may keep these unstable people away from work for 1 to 8 weeks. With psychotherapy these people should be returned to work as soon as possible and usually within 1 to 2 weeks. My feeling is that if possible they should be kept on the job. People with tensions and anxieties usually do much better while working although we should not carry this principle to an absurd degree. There are tense and anxious people who simply cannot work because of the severity of the physical symptoms.

POST-TRAUMATIC ENCEPHALOPATHY

Regardless of the severity of the head trauma, the pretraumatic personality of the employee usually determines in most cases the length of time off from work. Given a relatively sound personality with healthy motivation, the employee will return to work within 2 to 4 weeks, unless of course a basilar fracture was sustained. Those with a poor pretraumatic personality structure who sustained a very slight head trauma may want to be out many weeks, even up to 1 or 2 years. However, serious attempts at psychotherapy and at securing healthy motivations should be made. The compensation problem should be settled as quickly as possible and if necessary, a lump-sum settlement should be given as part of the therapy. The longer these people stay out of work, the harder it is to get them to return to work. We will meet with many resistances from the patient's relatives, the patient's lawyers and the patient's physician.

7. *The Placement and Management of Employees with Neurologic Disabilities*

IF EVERY MAN mended a man, then the whole world would be mended. In any work place, there will be among the employees those with a neurologic disease in various phases of the process. An enlightened management has realized that it is good business to hire the handicapped. A reservoir of skills rests with the physically and psychiatrically handicapped person and industry is beginning to realize that former fears of hiring them are unfounded and that industry needs these skills. The conservation and utilization of human resources of all kinds is vital to our country. The restoration of dignity to these people, the regaining of their self respect, the contribution that they can make to society through working are all part of the rewards of a rehabilitation program for the handicapped when there is a gainful occupation at the heart of the program.

These people invariably have a high desire to work. When properly placed, effectively supervised and adequately followed up by plant physicians, they are excellent and grateful workers. We must remember that each case has to be considered individually on its own merits.

In my work I have been familiar with a number of these neurologic conditions and I wish to mention a few of them and discuss what might be done in each case. The conditions which I shall discuss are as follows, viz.:

1. Multiple sclerosis
2. Epilepsy
3. Sciatic neuritis
4. Brachial neuritis
5. Hemiplegia and monoplegia
6. Retrobulbar and optic neuritis
7. Postoperative brain tumor
8. Amyotrophic lateral sclerosis
9. Subacute combined sclerosis
10. Progressive muscular dystrophy
11. Myotonia acquisita
12. Post-traumatic encephalopathy
13. Subarachnoid hemorrhage

MULTIPLE SCLEROSIS

Jobwise, there may be problems with employees who have multiple sclerosis. These can usually be surmounted if the members of the team who will be working with the employee have the desire to do so and if the company's policy is to hire the handicapped. One of the first problems to be met with is whether the employee knows that he has multiple sclerosis or not. When or even if to tell a patient he has multiple sclerosis is always a difficult decision to make. Some physicians feel strongly that the patient should never know what the diagnosis is but that some relative should know the diagnosis. I feel strongly that when an employee develops multiple sclerosis and is able to continue to work, though there may be relapses and repeated absences, that employee should know what the facts are. If he is to rehabilitate himself he should know what he has to face — what is ahead of him — because only then will he be able to plan effectively for the future. He should be told what there is to know about multiple sclerosis and he should be informed about the nearest chapter of the national multiple sclerosis association. He should be encouraged to join this chapter and attend its meetings and participate in its activities. Through association with other patients with the disease, through regular monthly meetings, reading the various publications such as the local chapter's bulletin of the publication of the national organization, engaging in the chapter's recreational, occupational and educational activities, he develops a useful psychological support for himself now and in the years to come.

Handicaps That May Have to be Considered in Placement and Management

1. Visual defects
2. Walking defects
3. Coordination defects
4. Stiffness and weakness of arms and legs
5. Speech defects
6. Personality problems
7. Co-worker problems

Visual Defects

Reduction in vision, blurring of vision, diplopia which may come and go from week to week, and nystagmus which may be marked from time to time, may call for placement on a job which does not demand much of the optic system. As an example, a person who formerly placed tiny screws into a part may be able to place a much larger unit into a larger part for the time being. Inspection may have to be changed from detailed to gross inspection temporarily. A patient may be able to do paper work temporarily in the department office instead of machine work. Ways can be found to keep these people working, though it may be more difficult in smaller industries.

Walking Defects

The person who has walked much on the job in the past may not be able to do so now because of ataxia, stiffness, weakness and poor coordination. A sitting job might be found temporarily until the relapse in symptoms recedes. I have known patients who have come to work in an auto, are carried to a wheel chair, and then wheeled into the plant for the day's work. Canes, crutches, etc. have been used by many of these people to get to work, to stay at work, and to do a day's work. These people are grateful for the opportunity to do something worthwhile, to accomplish something by themselves and they will always be thankful and loyal to those who have befriended them.

Coordination Defects

Ataxia due to posterior column involvement will hamper some individual's abilities to do their accustomed work especially if this work has been detailed, fine, fussy and needing a steady hand. The ataxia cannot be too great or objects cannot be held, even for gross inspection. Sometimes, a job might be found in another department in which case a temporary transfer might be made. After the plant physician has decided what the employee can and can not do and how he might do it and for how long, then the personnel department can go to work and find a suitable job for him.

Speech Defects

As a rule, speech defects in the form of slurred speech, explosive speech or ataxic speech will not interfere with work or with communication about work. If the patient can still write, he can still communicate with his supervisor. He can usually hear without any defects because it is rare to have multiple sclerosis affect the hearing mechanism. The effect of a speech defect on the co-workers of the employee with multiple sclerosis may be disarming at first, but if these co-workers have been properly and effectively oriented as to the goal of rehabilitation of the handicapped, this potential difficulty can be overcome.

Stiffness and Weakness of Arms and Legs

Since multiple sclerosis attacks various parts of the body at different times through involvement mainly of the cerebellar system, the optic system, the pyramidal tract system and the posterior column system producing deep sensory disturbances, various symptoms and signs will be produced at different times. The arms may be spastic and stiff and weak at one time while in another relapse, the arms may be very little involved while the legs may be spastic, weak and stiff. Therefore, the plant physician should follow these patients from time to time and follow up to see if the work situation is agreeable for that particular phase of the illness. The ability to do certain manual jobs or to walk much on the job will depend on the location of the pathology at any one given time and as to the severity of the process at that time. The supervisor should be appraised of this possibility so that he will be able to plan more effectively for the employee.

Personality Problems

Euphoria and elation have usually been described as common to the multiple sclerotic patient. In general this is true and this frame of mood certainly helps the patient to live from day to day. However, one may also see depressive moods and irritability. I have seen severe instances in which the patient is in a wheel chair and is severely disabled and yet he denied his inability to work at his former job. He overcompensated to his disability and became quite angry when he was told that he was unable to work anymore. In a way, this was fine for him as he was able to maintain his integrity and keep his defenses up, but this made it more difficult for all of us who had to deal with him and his work and home situation. These patients usually are cheerful and optimistic and will pitch in for work in a grand style. They will take orders readily and carry them out faithfully.

Co-worker Problems

The sight of disabled people will upset some persons. They might also become irritated at the extra time and attention that are given to these handicapped persons. Unless the co-workers are oriented properly by the supervisor or the plant physician as to how to behave, what to expect and what everybody in the plant is trying to do with these people, there may well be trouble. I have seen no difficulty where the soil has been prepared for the reception of these people back into the department or for the welcoming for the first time of a new employee with a handicap. The supervisor should be briefed by the plant physician about the condition and as to what the supervisor can expect in the way of work performance in the future. He should be told that there may be relapses during which the employee may be absent from work for a few weeks. The plant physician need not go into details about the illness but should give the supervisor enough information about the present status, the disabilities, and what the physician thinks that the patient might be able to do with safety to himself, to his co-workers, and to the plant. The supervisor then will be able to talk with the other members of his department about how they are going to accept the person with multiple sclerosis. A good general policy to follow in this respect is "Treat them as normal people." We do this same thing with employees returning from the mental hospital to a department. The other employees have a chance to talk this whole situation over with the supervisor, ask questions, and in general to get acquainted with the problem, to reduce anxiety thereby, and to develop a healthy attitude towards the handicapped person. *Most handicapped people don't want any favors.* They want to be treated like normal, average human beings. Problems will arrive inevitably wherever there are people working together, whether they are all healthy or not, but they can always be solved amicably and fairly when there is *"a heart in the department."*

In times of slack work, employees are laid off because of lack of suitable work. An employee with multiple sclerosis may be one of these employees to be laid off. Seniority usually rules this selection in most plants. However, when an employee with multiple sclerosis is affected by this rule, other factors should be considered. This employee may have been a marginal employee in that he had not worked too steadily because of absences due to relapses of his multiple sclerosis. In fairness to the afflicted and affected employee, the medical department might be able to place this man on sick leave so that he would be eligible to receive some salary from his sick benefit. We must realize that a person with multiple sclerosis is not wanted by most companies as a new employee and particularly in a time of economic recession. He will probably seek a new job but with the attitude of most companies today toward hiring a person with mulitple sclerosis, in spite of all the work that has gone on and is being done by the President's Committee for the Employment of the Physically Handicapped and the various Governor's committees of the various states, he does not have much of a chance to get a new job. The employee with multiple sclerosis must be placed on sick leave only on the merits of his individual case because a healthy person with the same seniority should not be penalized for being healthy. A problem such as this must be handled according to the policy of each company and also must be handled on an individual basis. However, wherever the handicapped person is, and whatever the handicap is, the company would do well to remember the words of that British philosopher who said about 400 years ago, "If every man mended a man, then the whole world would be mended."

Epilepsy

The patient with epilepsy is being accepted more widely by more companies for employment, and the employee who develops epilepsy is being retained by more companies, but there is still much education of employers to be done. The stigma of epilepsy, going back thousands of years, still hangs on in spite of medical and social enlightenment in this area and better medical treatment and handling of cases. The employees with epilepsy are charting a fine record of safety and productivity in those companies which accept them for employment, place them properly and follow them up periodically in the medical and industrial relations department. The supervisor plays a key role in the management of these employees. He should be given whatever medical facts are necessary for him to effectively manage his employee with epilepsy.

In a report entitled "The Person with Epilepsy at Work," the Committee on Psychiatry in Industry, Group for the Advancement of Psychiatry, makes the following comments, viz:

Estimates of the number of persons in the United States who suffer from convulsive seizures, commonly called epilepsy or fits range from 800,000 to 1,500,000. The President's Committee on the Physically Handicapped states that "Treatment of epilepsy with anticonvulsants results in complete control of seizures in over 50% of cases, a reduction of seizures to the extent that patients may be rehabilitated socially and vocationally in an additional 30% of the cases.

Despite this indication that the majority of epileptics are employable, there is considerable resistance in industry to their employment.

This lag between medical progress and society's rejection of a person with epilepsy is based on erroneous but long-standing attitudes about the person with seizures. There have always been fears, anxieties and misconceptions concerning individuals subject to sudden loss of consciousness and convulsions. A stigma has been attached to epilepsy for many centuries. Many people have believed the disease is inherited. This contributes to the social stigma of epilepsy. Laws in many states discriminate against the epileptic. It is because of such persistent misconceptions and anxieties that industry rejects many persons or discharges them.

In the light of modern medical advances these attitudes are unrealistic, actually wasteful of human resources, and specifically deprive industry of a sizable group of acceptable workers. In areas of labor shortage and in less popular occupations this potential of manpower supply cannot be profitably overlooked. Quite aside from these realistic gains in employee potential, industry cannot afford not to liberalize its policies toward epileptics. Faced with an applicant who reports having had seizures, the natural tendency of the employment officer is to refuse him. Uncertainty over a greater incidence of accidents, the possible disruption of the work group, and the stigma of the illness all combine to create a barrier against the epileptic. Confronted with a reported seizure of an employee, the most common reaction in industry is to dismiss him. This response, too, is understandable when questions of possible injury and compensation problems arise.

For these reasons many individuals subject to any type of seizure, feel they have to conceal this fact in order to secure employment. Certainly, the epileptic who tells the truth should not be penalized for it, yet this is often the case. It is obviously better for the employee and for the company to be in possession of all the facts of his handicap. In this way, safe placement plans can be carried out, based upon the recommendations and treatment of the employee's own physician and the judgement of the industrial physician. The result of refusing to employ or of indiscriminate firing of epileptics is to force the person who has seizures to conceal his problem. Many are therefore employed without industry's knowledge and are unwittingly assigned to jobs which are dangerous to themselves and to others. As a result both management and the worker are in a far greater jeopardy than they might be if this problem were handled in keeping with modern medical understanding.

Merely eliminating people who have had seizures prior to the time of hiring, were this possible, would still not be a solution to the problem since seizures can develop after a period of seizure-free employment. Even when a person has not experienced seizures before employment, there are many factors within and without industry which influence the development of such attacks. Head injury, brain tumor, toxic conditions, and arteriosclerosis are a few examples of these factors.

In the section of this same report titled *"Placement"* the committee made the following statements, viz:

Epileptics, like other people, vary and therefore a "blanket policy" is ineffective. The type of epilepsy, the seizure pattern, the presence or absence of an "aura," the time of day at which attacks may occur, all these and many more factors vary greatly from one individual to another so that it is impossible to generalize freely concerning the rules of placement of the epileptic.

However, there are some relevant general considerations. The aim is to protect the epileptic from hazardous situations where he may injure himself or others or damage equipment. Common types of environmental hazards are moving machinery, open electrical circuits, working at heights, and driving. Seizures may be precipitated by a wide variety of noxious substances. The most common protective policy has been the assigning of employees to jobs that are relatively free from hazard.

Usually, the work assignment is made on the basis of the employee's condition. It would be inadvisable for a person whose seizures have not been brought under conrtol, to engage in such activities as climbing or driving. The placement of an epileptic who has only occasional seizures, all of them during his sleep, would generally present no particular difficulty. He could work at heights under hazardous conditions.

In arriving at decisions regarding individual placement the period of trial employment becomes more important for the epileptic than for other handicapped employees. When considering the employment of a person with seizures such a probationary period offers opportunity for realistically evaluating the potential contributions the epileptic may be able to make to the company.

One occasional problem is the effect that a seizure has on other workers. Many find this a disturbing experience with a resultant loss of indeterminate amount of time and effective attention to the job at hand.

It is important to realize that the epileptic has the same assets and abilities as others and that his awareness of the fact that he is handicapped may result in his being a conscientious, careful and meticulous worker. In placing the epileptic, the thinking of those responsible should not be negatively expressed entirely in terms of the epileptic's liabilities; these may be overstressed, especially if many restrictions are considered on the basis of rather sweeping generalizations.

In the section titled, *The Function of the Plant Physician,* the committee stated as follows:

The industrial physician has the responsibility first of diagnosing the limitations and assets of each patient. This is facilitated by the maintenance of close liaison with the family physician and consultants. The next task of the industrial physician is the acquisition of thorough knowledge of the working conditions for each job. He then has the responsibility of suggesting to the Personnel Department the restrictions which may be required in the hiring, placement and transfer of these employees. Personnel workers then have the responsibility of the specific steps in the placement and transfer of these employees.

In addition to these functions the plant physician must also be responsible for the instruction of personnel who may come in contact with the epileptic. This group includes supervisors, the epileptic's co-workers and first-aid personnel. Emphasis in this instruction should be on the care of the worker during a convulsion and on appropriate. healthy behavior of those witnessing a convulsion. It is hoped that the latter task has been accomplished by educational, preventive measures. The care of a worker during a convulsion is, as noted above, one of injury prevention. Such care can be delegated to an emotionally mature person after a brief amount of instruction.

These tasks are those that ordinarily fall within the scope of activity of industrial physicians and are not, in general, any more demanding than their numerous other duties. The chief difficulty that industry encounters in this connection arises in small plants in which there is no resident physician. In such situations industry has as an alternative, the employing or maintaining in immediate accessibility someone trained in the handling of a post-seizure patient. This need not be a physician but can be a first-aid worker or nurse whose knowledge is sufficiently extensive to recognize a condition which is serious enough to warrant calling a physician. In the vast majority of seizures no such step is necessary.

There is very great need for a significant change in the general attitude toward the epileptic and his problems. This arises not only from a humane orientation toward the epileptic but from society's need to utilize the contributions that these people can make. Long-standing prejudices and beliefs must give way to a fresh, more realistic outlook compatible with the increased skill and knowledge in managing epilepsy. In these matters, the industrial physician can play a decisive role in working out methods of achieving a change of attitude that can benefit both industry and the epileptic.

In another section of this pamphlet, the committee declares that the Workmen's Compensation laws should be revised so that the second injury clause is applicable to epileptics.

I have spent some time discussing multiple sclerosis and epilepsy because these are the two main general neurologic conditions which one sees rather often in any industrial or occupational medical practice. To be sure, sciatic and brachial neuritis are also common but these conditions involve localized areas of the body and do not provoke such emotional overtones and they usually recover or become markedly improved. The psychological lift that patients with multiple sclerosis and epilepsy derive from employment is so great and lasting that everyone benefits. These patients should be followed regularly in the medical department so that the feelings, the attitudes, and the thoughts of the handicapped employee will be known in regard to the job situation and in regard to his own illness.

Sciatic Neuritis

Employees who develop the usual infectious and inflammatory type of sciatic neuritis may or may not have symptoms severe enough to warrant being absent from work. In the severe type, the patient may be away from his work for several weeks with restricted activity. The mild and moderate cases may or may not be able to continue on with their work. Some may continue with their regular work if it does not interfere too much with their neuritis and cause more pain and discomfort. A walking job may have to be changed temporarily to a sitting job. At times, a sitting job is too painful and a combination of sitting and walking may be found more comfortable. When these patients return to their jobs following an attack of sciatic neuritis, their legs may have to be protected temporarily. Their physician may desire that they work only half time for awhile — or vary their work from time to time to keep the sitting and the standing to a minimal.

If the neuritis is of the symptomatic type caused by a ruptured intervertebral disc or a degenerated disc, the recovery may be prolonged or only improved. A different job may have to be found permanently for these people. At times, wasting of the muscles of the afflicted leg occurs and a corresponding weakness develops in the course of a sciatic neuritis. In this case, a radical revision of the job may have to be made on the advice of the attending and plant physician.

Brachial Neuritis

When an employee returns to work following an attack of acute brachial neuritis, consideration may have to be given to his placement if there is still some pain and restriction of use of that arm. If the dominant arm was involved, then a job in which the other arm might be able to do some of the work might be found. An inspection job or a stock room job or a checking job might be practical. He may be able to work part time for awhile until the arm is completely healed. These conditions may take many weeks and months to heal and the employee becomes restless at home and wants to be doing something to keep his mind occupied. This placement at times takes much imagination and ingenuity but usually always pays off to the advantage of all concerned.

Hemiplegia and Monoplegia

Employees who have suffered a cerebral vascular accident often recover to the point where they are able to return to their former job or to one that they can manage. If mental deterioration is nonexistent or minimal, and the will to work is adequate, and motor and sensory recovery is sufficient so that a creditable job can be done, these patients can carry on for some time. I have had instances where the leg has recovered exceptionally well so that the patient could resume his former duties even though these entailed some walking (which was good physical therapy). An inspector, a time study man or a foreman could carry on if the dominant arm was not involved or if it had recovered sufficiently. Each case must be individualized and studied separately and recommendations for placement made by the attending and plant physician and carried out by the personnel department. I have had one middle aged patient who had 3 separate vascular accidents with almost complete recovery each time and he is still working 7 years after his first vascular accident and doing his usual creditable job. His spirits are still high and he is producing well. He has had 7 years of feeling useful to himself, to his family and to his company.

I have had 5 employees who have suffered a weakness of the dominant right arm in a cerebral vascular accident. Each recovered sufficiently to return to his former job, which entailed the use of that right arm. If walking was prominent in the job and only an arm was involved, work can go on when the acute phase is over. This keeps his mind occupied and active.

The following factors are important to consider in the placement of these persons, viz:

1. The policy of the company relative to taking back on the job employees who have had a neurologic disease. This involves the willingness of management at any level, to plan, to spend time, to invent, to improvise, and to work with the medical department in going all out to find a job or to alter jobs to fit the remaining abilities of the handicapped.

2. The type of job that the employee had before he became ill.

3. The demands of the job — physical, emotional and skilled factors.

4. The type of severity of the lesion and the remaining disability.

5. The personality of the patient before the accident and whether he has high or low motivation to work.

Retrobulbar and Optic Neuritis

Employees who are recovering from an attack of retrobulbar or optic neuritis may have impaired vision which might possibly affect their former working efficiency. Many of them will have a strong urge to return to work before their vision has completely recovered. If the attending eye physician consents to this idea after he and the plant physician have discussed the job, its demands, etc., then a suitable job might be found if the former one had too many demanding factors for vision. A job with more gross visual requirements may have to be found temporarily and he may have to take more "work breaks." As vision returns to normal or near normal, consideration of his returning to his former job must be constantly considered. If some degree of atrophy remains in either conditions then a job with lower visual requirements may have to be found on a permanent basis. Eye glasses with some magnification may assist the patient temporarily.

Postoperative Brain Tumor

Occasionally, an employee who has had an operation for the removal of a brain tumor, will have recovered motor power, sensation and mental faculties sufficiently to be considered for reemployment. If the tumor was completely removed as in the case of a meningioma, then the entire plan of the "return-to-work" program must be different from when the tumor was not completely removed as in the case of an infiltrating tumor. In the former instance, the program should be focused on the ultimate recovery of the employee and his return to his former job. Phases of the rehabilitation program wherein more demanding work can be developed from time to time can be planned with the constant advice of the plant physician and the attending neurosurgeon. The supervisor and the personnel department will always have to be counseled throughout the rehabilitation.

The rehabilitation of employees who have had an infiltrating tumor removed must be limited in the goal to be reached and in its scope. I have had a number of such people who have been able to work for many months and a few years following the original operation. It is true that irradiation and other therapy may continue and there may be relapses, but the psychological lift that these patients get from some worthwhile work is a joy to behold. Supervision at any level always feels rewarded in these cases even though it may be temporary. Hard work and imaginative thinking has been necessary to make jobs, and at times production has suffered temporarily. The histopathologic type of the tumor and its position and its rate of growth will determine whether there is any chance of the patient returning to work. We must be guided by the neurosurgeon. These unfortunate people are grateful for the extra months of respectable work and of associating once again with their co-workers.

Amyotrophic Lateral Sclerosis

With this disease I shall enter a field of degenerative conditions which are rare but which may produce certain phases of the process that allow the patient to work for months or years. Placement problems will develop and the medical management will need constant supervision.

Once I saw a 61 year old employee who had been referred to me because of increasing stiffness and weakness of his legs. He had worked 42 years for the company, had had 3 visits to the medical department in that time, had not missed a day of work from illness, and his medical record testified to this record by being paper thin. He now had amyotrophic lateral sclerosis affecting his legs which were stiff and weak, and there was a dragging of the right foot. His desire to continue to work was high, and he saw no reason not to work. I saw him about every two months for the next 4 years at which time he retired with normal retirement benefits and disability benefits. Fortunately, the neurologic process had not invaded extensively the cervical area of the spinal cord and he could still work rather well with his hands. He finally had to use two canes to get around. His job was changed to a completely sedentary one and he was shifted from an assembly line job to an inspection job. His knowledge and wisdom of the product made him an excellent inspector. He took physical therapy treatments at the office of an orthopedic surgeon near his home and felt that his legs felt better following treatments. His spirits were always high and contagious by virtue of his ever present smile and wonderful philosophy of life. Here was an instance where everybody concerned with the life and strife of one lone man pitched in and collaborated so that his remaining working years with the company could be worthwhile.

Subacute Combined Sclerosis

The problem that these patients present is one of weakness, stiffness, ataxia and incoordination of arms, hands, legs and feet of varying degrees. Adjustments in the work situation will depend on whether the pathologic process is more prominent in the cervical or lumbar areas of the spinal cord affecting either the upper or lower extremities and whether the pathologic process is more prominent in the pyramidal tract area or the posterior column area of the spinal cord. Ataxia will be less if the posterior column involvement is minimal. Spasticity and weakness will be less if the pyramidal tract involvement is minimal. One may see marked ataxia in the hands and fingers and very little spasticity while there may be marked spasticity and very little ataxia in the legs and feet. Pernicious anemia is quite often the cause of this neurologic condition. If the afflicted employee has the will to work and a job suitable for his reduced skills can be found in his or another department, all will benefit.

Progressive Muscular Dystrophy

This condition is rare in an occupational setting because of the rarity of the disease itself and by the fact that the disease process itself usually renders the sufferer incapable of performing any work early in the course of the illness. However, I have been following a 42 year old employee who has had the disease for many years and is still working. His work has had to be changed from time to time but he continues to do creditable work in spite of the weakness of certain groups of muscles. I cite this case as an illustration of what can be done in a seemingly chronic situation.

Myotonia Acquisita

A 26 year old male patient was referred to me in 1946 by one of the plant physicians because (1) he had trouble releasing his hold on anything he grasped, and (2) he could not speak fluently when he started to speak. The first complaint had made the performance of his duties in a field division maintenance unit very difficult because he had to climb poles, towers, buildings, scaffolding etc. in the course of his work and he couldn't let go easily. This slowed him up on his job and was a worry to the safety department if he ever got into an emergency situation. This condition had evidently developed originally in the army as I found out in questioning him, but at the time of discharge his complaints were so minimal that he paid no attention to them at that time. Following discharge and resuming his former prewar work the condition gradually became worse. At the time of reemployment following his discharge he said nothing of these complaints because he did not attach any significance to them. I placed him on quinine three times a day which helped him tremendously but we "grounded" him for his own safety and that of the others around him. He continues to work effectively at this date. He received a Veterans pension as he was able to prove service connection.

Post-traumatic Encephalopathy
(Post-traumatic Head Syndrome)

An employee who has suffered a head injury may return to work with a few lingering symptoms. These symptoms usually are not serious but may be annoying. A temporary job adjustment may be necessary because the employee may develop a headache or dizziness on bending over or during other sudden changes of body position. He may be able to work only half time for a few weeks because of tiredness, easy fatiguability and generalized weakness. This gradual return to work helps these people tremendously. A head injury of any type with or without unconsciousness usually brings various physical and emotional symptoms which may be of any severity and endure for a few days to a few months. They range from headache, dizziness, easy fatiguability, extreme tiredness, weakness, poor concentration, "sticky" thinking, tender areas of the head, numb feelings of the head and face, increased tension, anxiety, fears and worry over many things. Anxiety and fear about returning to work often delays the return to work. Also, the pre-accident personality of the employee and his desire to return to work will determine to a large extent if and when he will return to his job. Some employees have been emotionally unstable before the injury to the head but have managed to get along on a marginal basis. They have compensated just enough to get by in their on-the-job and off-the-job life. An injury to the head often is "the last straw" and the employee literally "falls apart" — in fact, he decompensates in varying degrees and a full blown neurosis develops. We should try extra hard to get these marginal employees back on the job as soon as possible to prevent fixation of symptoms, to reduce anxiety and fears about the job and to restore confidence and dignity to them. The longer they are out of work the greater the secondary gain. The head is a symbol of many different things to many different people. When it is injured, people imagine that all kinds of dire things will happen to them, viz: they will go crazy, their brain will soften, they will lose their memory, they will say silly things, their mind will get weak, they will lose control over their behavior, they will look funny, etc. We can reduce the possibilities of anxieties, doubts, fears and imaginations and useless worries by getting them back on the job as early as possible and by counseling them from time to time, so that their fears can be nipped in the bud early.

Employees who were emotionally stable before an injury to the head will usually return to work as soon as their physical condition permits them to do so. At times, they wish to return to work too soon and they must be urged to follow their attending physician's advice. They have accepted the head injury philosophically and in a mature way and if there is any emotional reaction it is usually minimal and accessible to intelligent handling.

Subarachnoid Hemorrhage

An employee who has recovered from an attack of subarachnoid hemorrhage may be able to return to work of some kind if the residual disability is not too great. Adjustments may have to be made as were done in the following case, viz:

A married man, aged 43 with 2 teenage children suffered a subarachnoid hemorrhage with involvement of the left thalamus in the pathologic process. This occurred in March, 1954 and left him with a right spastic hemiparesis and a disagreeable sensation of the right face, arm, body and leg, described by him variously as burning, a tightness, a heaviness, "as if the right side is in a cast," "my right face feels like a hot flash all the time," etc. He improved to the point where he could walk with a limp and use the right arm fairly well. He wanted to return to work in July, 1954. We agreed that he could do so from a physical viewpoint. He had been a toolmaker before the vascular accident but he could not do this work at this time. He was given a job of inspection of screws and other machine parts. He returned to work half time in August, 1954 and full time in September, 1954. After a year of this work he was placed on a clerical job for about 4 years. Here, he checked blueprints, ordered bushings and other material and he performed well. Then, because of department reorganization he went into the tool crib about 2 months ago as a helper on a temporary basis. I have seen him every 3 months and he has done well, feels that he is really accomplishing something. Now, 6 years after this cerebral vascular accident, this man is still working, doing a job and supporting his family. It has been worth it.

8. Trauma to the Central and Peripheral Nervous Systems

THE CENTRAL NERVOUS SYSTEM and the peripheral nerves are injured by trauma and external toxic agents sufficiently often enough to warrant a discussion of the topic.* I shall divide the discussion into four parts, viz: (1) injuries of the brain and its coverings; (2) injuries of the spinal cord and its coverings; (3) injuries of the peripheral nerves; (4) physical and chemical agents and their reactions on the central and peripheral nervous systems.

Injuries of the Brain and Its Coverings

A list of the more common conditions in this category is as follows:
1. Concussion of the brain and fracture of the skull.
   - (a) traumatic epilepsy
   - (b) delayed apoplexy
   - (c) traumatic encephalitis
   - (d) abscess
   - (e) meningitis
   - (f) cysts of the brain
   - (g) arachnitis
   - (h) serous meningitis
2. Traumatic meningeal hemorrhage.
3. Subdural hematoma.
4. Spontaneous meningeal hemorrhage.
5. Postconcussion syndrome.
6. Post head trauma personality conditions.
7. Electric shock to central nervous system.
8. Compressed air illness.

Injuries of the Spinal Cord and Its Coverings

1. Fractures and dislocations of the spine, gunshot and stab wounds.
2. Hematomyelia.
3. Herniation of the intervertebral disc.
4. Concussion of the spinal cord.

Injuries of the Peripheral Nerves

1. Traumatic injury.
2. Toxic injury.

Physical and Chemical Agents and Their Reaction on the Central and Peripheral Nervous System

---

* Some of this chapter has been modified for this monograph from *Injuries of the Brain and Spinal Cord and their Coverings*, ed. 3, by Brock, and from *A Textbook of Clinical Neurology*, ed. 8, by Israel Wechsler.

INJURIES OF THE BRAIN AND ITS COVERINGS

Concussion of the Brain and Fracture of the Skull

Occupational physicians should be familiar with the symptoms and signs of concussion of the brain because head injuries do occur at the work place, especially in industry. Although the injured employees are transferred to a community hospital immediately in most instances, the physician should be able to make a tentative diagnosis at the work place. A concussion may occur following a direct blow to the head or following an explosion near the head. The blow may be severe or light. Instances are on record in which the blow was severe, but there was no fracture of the skull and no damage to the brain. On the other hand, a blow may be very light and the brain damage very severe, and the skull fractured. The symptoms and signs of the condition following a head injury depend on the type of blow, the direction and intensity of the blow, the type, location and extent of the skull fracture when present, and the amount of damage done to the brain. The patient's condition also depends on whether the fracture was simple or compound. If infection occurs later, this also alters the course of the illness, but the occupational physician would probably not care for the patient at this stage as the patient would be in a community hospital. A few general rules to follow in sizing up a head injury are as follows, viz:

Head Injury Diagnostic Reminders

1. If a fracture occurs, consciousness is usually disturbed at once — from momentary loss to profound coma, and at times death.
2. Usually, there is some disturbance of consciousness.
3. Signs and symptoms of concussion may occur after a variable duration.
4. Usually, the symptoms and signs of concussion appear in direct proportion to the intensity of the blow and the extent of the fracture.
5. Coma will be deep if there is edema or bleeding within the skull from brain or meningeal tearing, which results in brain compression.
6. Respirations will be deep and stertorous and often Cheyne Stokes.
7. The pulse will be slow and full.
8. The face will be flushed.
9. The feet will be cold.
10. Bleeding from the mouth, nose or ears.
11. Presence of cranial nerve palsies.
12. Escape of cerebrospinal fluid.
13. Depression at the site of injury.

14. The pupils will at first be contracted, then dilated. The pupil on the side of the injury will often be dilated and fixed.

15. Ecchymoses will occur about the eyes, mastoid and back of the neck.

Prognosis

1. Varies with the severity and location of the injury.
2. Death occurs in many cases.
3. Fractures of the base are more serious than those of the vault.
4. Depressed and comminuted fractures are worse than simple fissured fractures.
5. Compound fractures increase the possibility of infection, abscesses and meningitis.
6. Fractures of the skull are serious both immediately and in the long run because even if the patient survives, he rarely recovers his preaccident intellectual, emotional and behavior level.
7. Recovery takes months or years and neurologic complications may be permanent, such as cranial nerve palsies, deafness and optic atrophy.

Treatment

1. Estimate the extent of the skull and brain damage.
2. Keep patient warm and administer sedatives to keep patient quiet. Morphine should probably not be used if basilar fractures are present as the medulla will be embarrassed sufficiently enough from hemorrhage and edema. Narcotics depress the medullary centers of respiration and circulation.
3. X-ray the skull with stereoscopic views.
4. Transfer to a hospital at once. If this is impossible and surgery is to be done in the plant surgery, then the surgeon will proceed to relieve brain pressure from depressed skull fragments and clean the wound with a thorough débridement.
5. Fluids intravenously as needed will be given.
6. Reassurance and support.

The patient will usually be transferred to a community hospital by the time a diagnosis of fracture of the skull and severe concussion is made. If the patient survives the first few hours, a return of consciousness, vomiting, headaches, and dizziness occurs. Various cranial nerve palsies might develop depending on the site of the injury. Jacksonian convulsions also may appear, along with focal symptoms and signs no different from any other cerebral lesion. Meningeal irritation may develop. Infection may occur in the later stage of this process from the infected materials, hair, etc. that have been driven into the brain through the fracture of the skull. Localized abscesses, small or large, superficial or deep may occur. Various mental states may develop from excitement to apathy, delirium, etc. Headaches, dizziness and ringing of the ears may also appear. Meningeal hemorrhage, traumatic encephalitis, traumatic epilepsy, delayed apoplexy, superficial or deep abscesses, infectious meningitis, serous meningitis, all may develop weeks or months later. Subdural hematoma also may appear weeks or months later.

Simple Concussion of the Brain

In simple concussion without fracture or compression, the following are reminders:

1. Momentary clouding of consciousness, a dazed feeling, or a real temporary loss of consciousness.

2. Headache at the site of the injury or at the occiput will be present.

3. Apathy, irritability, poor memory, poor concentration and mental dullness may be present.

4. Dizziness is usually present and annoying.

5. Other symptoms as insomnia, weakness, poor appetite, sweating, labile pulse, depression or excitability, and inability to work may occur.

6. The above symptoms may occur at once or they may appear weeks or months later.

7. Personality may be changed and this may depend on the preaccident personality makeup of the person injured and on the severity of the injury.

8. The emotional overlay of many of the symptoms makes it difficult to estimate whether the symptoms are a result of the injury or are psychogenic.

9. The compensation situation complicates the problem of diagnosis because a factor of motivating secondary gain is introduced into the picture.

Prognosis

1. Difficult to evaluate because of the factors of the personality of the injured employee and the compensation element.

2. Is good for complete recovery if there has been no prolonged period of unconsciousness, no depression of the brain and no psychological factors involved.

3. Most cases recover from the immediate injury but the ultimate recovery is in doubt because of the above factors.

Treatment

1. Rest in bed with no bathroom privileges. This can be gauged in direct proportion to the period of unconsciousness. At least a week in bed should be insisted on if there were only momentary unconsciousness — more if unconsciousness were longer.

2. Estimate extent of damage by means of: (1) neurologic examination; (2) x-rays of the skull with stereoscopic views will be taken depending on condition of patient; (3) close observation; and (4) hospitalization should be considered in most cases and especially when unconsciousness is present.

3. Sedatives to keep the patient quiet. Narcotics should not be given because of the depressive effects on the medullary centers of respiration and circulation.

4. When depression of the skull does not clinically seem to be present and when there are no signs of meningeal hemorrhage, the patient may be allowed more freedom in bed.

5. Lumbar puncture should not be done in most cases. Some physicians feel that a lumbar puncture might be done to relieve intracranial pressure if the headache is severe. However, in the author's opinion, intracranial pressure usually builds up higher following a lumbar puncture than it was previously.

6. Symptomatic treatment with good nursing care.

7. Psychotherapy should be started from the time of injury and should be part of the intelligent management of the patient. The seeds of future traumatic compensation neurosis begin to be sown as soon as the patient awakens from his unconsciousness and begins to survey and assess his situation. Effective management at this stage may prevent the development of a traumatic neurosis, and if convalescence seems to be unduly prolonged because symptoms of headache, dizziness, weakness, tiredness, etc. continue or/and the desire to get well and get back to work seems to be weak, the physician should begin to look for emotional and personality factors and the possibility of secondary gain. This could be the time to call in a psychiatrist — at an *early* stage rather than after 1 to 3 years of compensation hearings.

8. Any litigation or compensation problem should be settled as quickly as possible before fixation of symptoms develops, but not before maximum recovery has been reached.

9. Alcohol should be forbidden in the convalescent stages. The patient will find out later, if he does drink, that usually his alcoholic capacity is severely limited following a head blow.

Occupational physicians usually see employees with simple concussion immediately following the injury. A diagnosis is made and the patient is usually transferred to a hospital for further observation and treatment. At times, the employee may be transferred to his home if his condition warrants. At any rate, the occupational physician will have an opportunity to follow through on the course of the injury. The injured employee will probably have his own family physician and probably a surgeon to care for him when he is in the hospital or at home. Nevertheless, the occupational physician should continue to show interest in the employee by making visits at the hospital or home. This keeps the occupational physician informed as to what is going on and it gives the injured employee the feeling that the company doctor and the company do care what happens to him. The relatives of the injured employee also need attention and some interpretations and explanation of the illness and the occupational physician can render a great service in many ways and relieve many anxieties of the relatives. He should, of course, keep in touch with the family physician and any other attending physicians. The occupational physician can also see if the family needs any assistance while the breadwinner is recovering. Any family needs help in times of unexpected accident and the company can always assist in many little ways. As the patient recovers and gets about, postconcussion symptoms may develop and the industrial physician should be familiar with this complication. I shall discuss this below.

Major Late Complications of Skull Fracture and Brain Injury

A. TRAUMATIC EPILEPSY

1. Convulsions, generalized or localized, may occur months or years following an injury. The injury usually is a severe brain injury with fracture of the skull. However, one occasionally sees convulsions following a minor head injury with no skull fracture and short period of unconsciousness.

2. Epileptic equivalents may occur, such as fainting, cyclic alterations of the personality, or irritability of temper, together with petit mal episodes.

3. Twilight states and narcolepsy may develop.

Treatment

1. Neurosurgical consultation for evaluation of advisability of operation for removal of epileptogenous focus.

2. Anticonvulsant therapy.

3. Psychotherapy.

4. Job placement.

B. DELAYED APOPLEXY

1. Acute cerebral hemorrhage may occur a few days or few weeks following the head injury producing the usual spastic weakness of arms and legs and weakness of the face.

2. Cerebral arteriosclerosis has *usually* been present before the cerebral hemorrhage — so that the injury is only a precipatating cause.

Treatment

1. Usual treatment for cerebral hemorrhage, viz.: bed rest, sedatives, intravenous fluids, coagulants, etc.

Prognosis

1. Depends on the locations and extent of the hemorrhage.
2. Death occurs in most instances.
3. If the patient survives the initial hemorrhage, there will be a residual of spastic hemiplegia with varying degrees disability. Other hemorrhages may occur in the future, one of which may be fatal.

C. TRAUMATIC ENCEPHALITIS

1. When present, the symptoms are similar to those of encephalitis of other causes, viz: altered mental state, varying degrees of unconsciousness, headache, nausea, vomiting, fever, apathy, somnolence, irritability, focal signs and symptoms of cortical irritation, etc., cranial nerve palsies, etc.

Treatment

Supportive — fluids intravenously, sedatives.

Prognosis

Guarded — depending of severity or the encephalitis process residuals of cranial nerve palsies, altered personality, mental states, etc. may occur.

D. BRAIN ABSCESS

Brain tumor may be suspected, but with a history of a previous brain injury, brain abscess must be considered.

1. Symptoms and signs depend on location, size of abscess and time interval between injury and onset of symptoms.
2. General symptoms and signs of an expanding intracranial lesion will occur, such as: local or general headache, anorexia, nausea, vomiting, visual symptoms of blurring, fever, leukocytosis, dizziness, nerve palsy, papilledema, neck rigidity, apathy, irritability.
3. Focal symptoms and signs will occur as the abscess grows, viz.: weaknesses of limbs, facial muscles, Jacksonian and generalized convulsions, contralateral sensory changes, reflex changes.
4. Fever and other general signs of infection may be present.

Treatment

1. Neurosurgical consultation.
2. Neurosurgical exploration or administration of antibiotics first to determine if the suspected abscess will respond to medicinal treatment.

Prognosis

1. Depends on response to medicinal or/surgical therapy.

E. MENINGITIS

1. History of previous brain injury.

2. Weeks after the injury, symptoms and signs of meningeal irritation will occur, viz: neck stiffness, headache, nausea, vomiting, fever, increased pulse rate, leukocytosis.

3. Lumbar puncture will be positive for increased leukocytes and organisms may be recovered from the spinal fluid.

Treatment

1. Usual meningitis therapy such as antibiotics, intravenous fluids and general supportive therapy, sedatives.

Prognosis

1. Guarded. Depends on effectiveness of antibiotic therapy.

F. CYSTS OF THE BRAIN

Mentioned but rarely seen.

G. ARACHNITIS

Mentioned but rarely seen.

H. SEROUS MENINGITIS

Mentioned but rarely seen.

Traumatic Meningeal Hemorrhage

1. May occur following any blow to the head, with or without fracture.

2. Hemorrhage may occur from arteries, veins, or sinuses and may develop at site of injury or on the opposite side from the injury *(contre coup)*.

3. Bleeding may be epidural or subarachnoid, on the vertex or base of skull.

4. The middle meningeal artery is the most common meningeal vessel to bleed.

5. Course of events is typical for this condition, viz.:

    a. Short period of unconsciousness or a dazed condition.

    b. Patient seems recovered and usually resumes his activities.

    c. After a few hours or a day or so, patient becomes somnolent, drowsy and stuperous.

    d. (1) Slow pulse; (2) Cheyne-Stokes or stertorous respiration; (3) Fever may be present, focal or generalized convulsion, weakness of the arm or/and leg develops; (4) papilledema; (5) ipsilateral pupil dilated; (6) contralateral corneal reflex lost; (7) aphasia develops early in left sides lesions; (a) symptoms may indicate a contralateral lesion (opposite to side of injury) if brain is pushed to opposite side of skull; (8) spinal fluid shows no blood, but may be yellow.

Treatment

1. Neurosurgical intervention to stop the bleeding.

Subdural Hematoma

1. Diagnosis difficult.
2. May follow fracture of the skull.
3. Caused by successive, continuous bleeding, inflammation and thickening of the inner dural surface. Soon a circumscribed thick mass of clot is formed, which acts like a tumor.
4. Develops a few weeks or months following a head injury.
5. Onset usually gradual — may be rapid, even apoplectic.
6. Neck rigidity may be marked.
7. Headache, vomiting, delirium, contralateral convulsions, paralysis of one or both limbs, papilledema develops.
8. Percussion tenderness of head usually marked.
9. Stupor, coma develop with remissions and relapses.
10. Cerebrospinal fluid usually yellow.

Treatment

1. Neurosurgical — to remove the hematoma.

Prognosis

1. Death occurs if undiagnosed.
2. Following removal of hematoma, patient may recover completely.

Note: 1. Subdural hematoma may develop in the following conditions, viz: chronic alcoholism, general paresis, senile dementia, scurvy, purpura, hemophilla, leukemia, the exanthemata, pertussis, and cerebral birth injuries.

Traumatic and Spontaneous Hemorrhage

1. May follow a mild head trauma without fracture.
2. Aneurysm of the brain may be present before the trauma and bleeding precipitated following the head trauma.
3. Brain and meningeal laceration and contusion without fracture will cause subarachnoid hemorrhage. Ventricular hemorrhage may also occur.
4. Headache is the first symptom — acute or subacute onset.
5. Alterations in consciousness from drowsiness to coma.
6. Vomiting may occur.
7. Convulsions may occur at any time of the process.
8. Neck is stiff, pupils may be unequal, deep reflexes may be absent.

9. Fever, slow pulse, leukocytosis may be present.

10. Focal cranial nerve signs may be present — especially if the bleeding comes from the area of the circle of Willis (aneurysm or bleeding) vessel, such as; ocular palsies, and ptosis.

11. Hemiplegia may occur if there is cerebral bleeding — this may occur following the meningeal picture.

12. With hemiplegia, there may be contralateral hyperreflexia, Babinski, choked disc and retinal hemorrhages.

13. Spinal fluid will be bloody — days later, the spinal fluid will be xanthochromie. Diagnosis is usually made by lumbar puncture.

Treatment

1. Bed rest, sedatives, hypnotics, and general supportive therapy, vitamin K and coagulants, viz., Dicumerol.

2. Neurosurgical consultation — angiography usually is done as soon after the rupture as the patient's condition warrants. This will localize the bleeding and determine cause. Surgery, such as tying off the common carotoid artery or other measures may save the patient's life.

Prognosis

1. Death may occur rapidly after the onset.

2. If diagnosis is made early enough and surgery performed successfully many patients can be saved.

3. Where surgery is not or cannot be performed, occasionally the patient may recover. About 30 per cent of patients die from the initial rupture. They may die later in the second or third attack of bleeding.

4. Focal signs may clear completely when the patient recovers or residuals may develop.

5. Various mental states may develop as residuals, especially the Korsakoff syndrome.

Remarks

1. Subarachnoid hemorrhage may also develop from the following causes: scurvy, periarteritis nodosa, bacterial endocarditis, hemophilia, leukemia, uremia, meningitis and hypertension.

Postconcussion Syndrome

1. Follows the immediate symptoms of concussion.

2. May be based on small punctate hemorrhage in the brain with gliosis.

3. Symptoms may last for weeks, months or years, but usually clear up.

4. Emotional overlay may be present in varying degrees.

5. The compensation factor. whether in industrial or nonindustrial accidents such as auto accidents, always plays a variable role in the course.

6. Usual symptoms are: headache, dizziness, weakness, easy fatigue-ability, photophobia, poor concentration, poor memory, irritability, mental dullness, noises in the ear, nausea, vomiting, tremors, insomnia, poor appetite.

Treatment

1. Sedatives or tranquilizers, hypnotics, analgesics. The author has found that Daprisal or Edrisal helps these patients to feel better by lifting their depressive spirits, reducing their headaches. These can be used in conjunction with tranquilizers.

2. Psychotherapy — very important. Allow the patient to ventilate as there are usually many personal, family and business problems to be discussed.

3. Early settlement of any claim.

Prognosis

1. Very difficult to state. With adequate and effective care early in the course and continued regular care with much emphasis placed on psycho-therapy in the later stages, much can be done with most of these patients. However, there is a small percentage of patients who have a chronic post-concussion syndrome which never seems to get better. The emotional factors loom large in these cases. The injury may have been a wonderful escape from the day's troubles and the patient will not give up the symptoms readily.

Post Head Trauma Personality Conditions

1. Personality alterations of all types may occur following a head trauma of any degree — from increased irritability to frank psychoses.

2. Pretrauma personality has always to be considered in evaluating the posttrauma personality.

3. The foreman, the employees' colleagues, his wife and children and his social friends all may notice the change and have difficulty in getting along with the employee.

4. Conferences with the employee at work, by his foreman, the industrial relations department, the industrial physician and talks with his wife all help to solve the problem. The team approach is effective.

5. Psychotherapy, tranquilizers, other sedatives, hypnotics, etc. should be used when indicated.

6. Although job transfers should be sparingly used, occasionally, a different job, with less pressure, less responsibility, etc. may be temporarily found for the employee.

7. Admission to a private mental hospital or a short period of treatment might be indicated. In seriously mentally ill patients, commitment to a mental hospital may be necessary.

Electric Shock to Central Nervous System

1. Death at once from sufficiently strong current.
2. Alternating currents more dangerous than direct.
3. *If not death,* sudden unconsciousness, convulsions, localized or general, slow pulse, vomiting, paralyses, headache, numbness, weakness, dizziness, loss of memory, delusions and hallucinations and depression.
4. *Treatment* — hospitalization at once.

Compressed Air Illness (Caisson Disease)

1. Due to sudden return to lower pressures, circulatory changes occur in spinal cord and brain.
2. Symptoms as pain in legs, arms, back and pit of stomach, has to double up (the bends), paralysis of legs of varying degree, sensory disturbances, urinary difficulties, headache, diplopia, convulsions, confusion and unconsciousness.
3. *Treatment* — hospitalization at once.

INJURIES OF THE SPINAL CORD AND ITS COVERINGS

In industry, injuries to the back will occur, which may produce spinal cord injuries. The major conditions which industrial physicians may encounter are as follows:

Fractures, Dislocations and Other Injuries

1. Important factor is the location and degree of injury to the spinal cord, meninges and the spinal roots.
2. A severe vertebral injury may have no spinal cord or spinal root injury. On the other hand, when there are very few signs of vertebral injury, the spinal cord and roots may be severely affected.
3. Tearing, crushing, severing of the cord, edema of and hemorrhage into the cord, tearing of the spinal roots and meninges, and compression of the cord may result in any injury.
4. Onset is rapid, usually immediately following the injury. The damage is done at the time of the injury. Occasionally, latent hemorrhage or a slow secondary compression may occur but this is rare.
5. The patient may die very shortly, the condition may remain stationary, and at times there is partial or complete recovery.
6. Symptoms and signs develop as follows: shock (usually no unconsciousness), motor paralysis of the extremities, sensory disturbances (complete or partial), below the level of the lesion and disorders of the sphincters.
7. Later, symptoms and signs of ascending and descending cord degeneration develop. General symptoms develop such as infections of the

bladder and kidneys, bed sores, general toxic symptoms, etc. — all of which have to be prevented if possible and treated when present.

8. Dislocations occur usually in the cervical region and result from blows and falls on the head, unusual stretching of the neck or bending of the head and neck. The dislocation may reduce itself but the cord injury will remain permanent.

9. Fractures occur more often in the low cervical, lower dorsal and upper lumbar regions.

10. Explosions, through sudden air compression, may cause spinal cord damage of varying degrees. Symptoms will depend on extent of cord damage. Gunshot wounds usually cause fracture of the spine and the bone fragments and the bullet may or may not cause cord symptoms depending on location of these foreign bodies.

11. Hemisection of the cord may be caused by gunshot or stab wounds. This is referred to as the Brown-Sequard syndrome.

12. High cervical injuries may produce the following: flaccid quadriplegia, possibly dyspnea, temperature rise, slow or rapid pulse, nystagmus, pupillary disturbances, hypothermia, fall in blood pressure and choked disc. In atlas and axis injuries, death occurs soon. In third and fourth cervical injury, the phrenic nerves may be involved and death occurs soon.

13. *Cervical enlargement injuries* may produce the following: pain in the arms if the spinal roots are involved, a Horner syndrome (lower cervical and upper thoracic).

14. *Thoracic injuries* may produce the following: paraplegia, occasional gastric dilatation, paralytic ileus and meteorism. Lower thoracic and upper lumbar injuries may produce lumbosacral root symptoms plus the cord injury.

15. *Cord injuries* produce at first flaccid paralysis, absent reflexes, and sphincter disturbances (first retention, then incontinence). In less severe cord injuries, the paralysis becomes spastic and the reflexes return.

Diagnosis

1. Depends on history of injury to the back, the sudden onset of spinal cord symptoms and the evidences of injury, x-rays of the spine help in the diagnosis. Lumbar puncture may show blood and in compression, may show a block.

Prognosis

Grave. Depends on location and extent of injury. In high cervical lesions death is usually rapid. In severe cord injury such as transection, tearing, etc., death usually occurs from infection of the kidney and bed sores. Residuals occur in the milder cord injuries such as weakness of the legs, sensory disturbances, spastic reflexes. Usually, there is no further improvement after a few weeks. Dislocations have a better prognosis as a rule.

Treatment

In industrial accidents, a diagnosis should be made at once with the aid of x-rays. The patient should then be transferred to a hospital as soon as possible. Medical and surgical care then will follow.

INJURIES OF THE PERIPHERAL NERVES

Industrial accidents often cause peripheral nerve injuries. Various operations, by their very nature, may produce neuropathies. The industrial physician should be aware of certain facts about these matters which would allow him to make a diagnosis, to refer to a consulting neurologist for further observation and treatment and to be ready, if necessary, to carry out certain physical therapy modalities. For further knowledge of these matters, the industrial physician is referred to textbooks on peripheral nerve injuries or/and neurology.

Reminders

1. *In complete interruption* of a nerve, the following occurs at once:
   a. Immediate and complete paralysis of muscles supplied by nerve.
   b. Soft and flabby muscles — no tone.
   c. Deep reflexes lost.
   d. Nerves and muscles not tender.
   e. Atrophy develops quickly.
   f. Pain is absent.
   g. No sensation below interruption.
   h. Area involved may feel cold.
   i. Trophic and vasomotor changes minimal.
2. *In Compression of a nerve* the following occurs:
   a. Partial paralysis of muscles supplied by nerve.
   b. Partial sensory disturbance in intensity and extensity.
   c. Atrophy not so severe and partial muscle tone is present.
   d. Mild vasomotor and trophic disturbances.
   e. If compression deepens, above symptoms increase. If compression decreases, above symptoms decrease.
   f. Delayed compression (from callous formation, sclerosing fibrous tissue, deformities, etc.) may occur months and at times a year after original injury. Best example is delayed ulnar palsy following an elbow fracture and subsequent cubitus valgus deformity and angulation of the ulnar nerve as it courses posterior to medial condyle.

g. *Tinel sign* occurs when a peripheral nerve is tapped and numbness is experienced in the peripheral end of the nerve. This usually means regeneration is occurring.

3. *In mild lesions of a motor and sensory nerve* the following occur:

a. *Signs of Irritation* such as intense pain from varying stimuli and often occurring spontaneously, hyperalgesic skin, which may be glossy and scaly, with nails that show trophic changes, with bizarre sensations.

b. Muscle tone not impaired much — firm muscles.

c. Atrophy varies.

4. *Causalgia*

a. Severe burning pains in area involved. Hyperesthesia severe — even air is disturbing.

b. Lesion may have been slight and no obvious evidence of paralysis, sensory loss, vasomotor or trophic changes. In other lesions, trophic and vasomotor changes do occur.

c. Median and sciatic nerves are common nerves affected.

d. Pain is paroxysmal — elicited often by motion.

e. Syndrome is probably sympathetic in nature.

f. Treatment is nonspecific and difficult.

5. *Regeneration* of axis cylinders produces formications, firming of muscles, trophic changes recede, sensory loss area diminished, electrical activity returns.

Tinel sign is the presence of tingling below a peripheral nerve lesion which has partially interrupted the nerve impulses. This is produced by tapping the nerve lightly with a percussion hammer. It is a good test to remember when one is not sure whether the nerve has been interrupted structurally (cut in two) complete or partially by compression by callus, bone splinter, etc. In complete section of the nerve, the numbness is absent above and below the lesion — in partial interruption from compression, the numbness is present both above and below the lesion.

Prognosis

1. Depends on type of injury, location, severity, medical and surgical treatment.

2. Partial nerve interruptions heal quicker than complete interruptions.

3. Early surgical treatment yields best results.

4. Recovery is slow — axon regeneration proceeds 1 to 2 mm. a day.

Treatment

1. Surgical for complete interruption, neuroma, compression of a nerve by scar tissue, callous, etc.

2. Antibiotics for infection.

3. Physical therapy (whirlpool bath, infrared, short wave diathermy, massage, exercises) for neuropathies caused from minor injuries, bruises, industrial operations, procedures, pressure, etc.

4. Medicinal therapy — vitamin B_1, B_{12}, analgesics, etc.

Ischemic Paralysis (Volkmann's)

1. Due probably to vascular disturbances, viz.: closure of large arteries by ligature or thrombosis and to rupture of vessels during an injury, occasionally too tight bandaging.
2. Circulatory and vasomotor factors are prominent.
3. The following changes occur, viz.: edema, cyanosis, fibrosis, sclerosis of muscles, skin, tendons, nail changes, skin color changes and extremity becomes hard.
4. No peripheral or segmental nerve disturbances.
5. Distal portion involved more than proximal.
6. Superficial sensation diminished.
7. Pain is always present.
8. Treatment is ineffectual.

Plexus Injuries

A. BRACHIAL

1. A wound above clavicle — upper and middle trunks and their nerves involved.
2. A wound below clavicle — cords and their derivations involved.
3. Axillary wounds are more apt to involve nerve trunks and blood vessels.
4. Upper plexus injuries — shoulder and upper arm involved chiefly. Sensory changes may be greater than motor changes.
5. In lower plexus injuries, the hand and forearm suffer most.
6. Entire plexus injuries:
   a. Wounds of the brachial plexus produce a temporary loss of function of the entire arm.
   b. Degree of damage can be assessed only after acute phase has passed.
   c. After about 2 weeks if the arm is paralyzed and anesthetic up to about C4, a complete brachial plexus palsy is present.
7. Upper arm type of paralysis (Duchenne-Erb):
   a. Due to injuries to 5th and 6th cervical roots (upper primary trunk).
   b. Causes of injuries — blows on the head pushing head away from shoulder or pushing shoulder down, resulting in tearing or stretching of roots, tumors, stab and gunshot wounds, fracture of clavicle, breech and vertex deliveries, cervicle rib.
   c. Results of injuries — paralysis of abduction, outward rotation of arm and elbow flexion, sensory disturbance on outer side of arm, biceps reflex lost, severe pain, vasomotor and trophic disturbances.
   d. Treatment, supportive, sedatives, analgesics, sling for weak arm, hospital for treatment and surgery if needed.
8. Lower arm type of paralysis (Klumpke-Dejerine):
   a. Due to injuries to 8th cervical and 1st dorsal roots (lower primary trunk).

b. Causes of injuries — above plus dislocations and fractures of head of humerus with overly ambitious attempts at reduction of such dislocations, quick stretching of arm upward, breech extractions.

c. Results of injuries — paralysis of hand flexors and small hand muscles, claw hand occurs occasionally, sensory disturbances on inner side of arm, Horner's syndrome occasionally occurs, pain, vasomotor and trophic disturbances.

d. Treatment — supportive, sedatives, analgesic, transfer to hospital for treatment of wounds and surgery if needed.

e. Atrophy sets in after a few weeks — a fact which aids in the diagnosis of complete plexus palsy.

PHYSICAL AND CHEMICAL AGENTS

Inorganic Compounds

Lithium and bromides are known to produce alterations in the psychic behavioral patterns following cumulative intoxication. Chronic exposure to high levels of fresh manganese oxide has produced a picture of basal ganglia damage. Copper may be involved in injury to the basal ganglia, i.e. Wilson's Disease. Thallium has produced damage to peripheral and central nervous systems in acute and subacute intoxications. Toxic encephalopathy has been reported in children with lead intoxication and with mercury intoxication in both children and adults. Mercury intoxication, of course, has been found to produce psychic changes early in the syndrome of intoxication. Arsenic has also been implicated as an agent capable of producing cerebral damage in chronic doses, probably due to vascular damage. Boron has been known to produce an encephalopathy, usually following acute or subacute exposures to boric acid or boron hydrides.

Organometallic Compounds

The organometallic compounds are more apt to produce encephalopathy than their inorganic-metal counterparts. This relates to the increased ability of organic-metallics to penetrate the cell. This is a function of their decreased polarity and general lipid solubility. Amongst this group, the organic tins, tetraethyl lead, organic arsenic, bismuth, and organo-mercury compounds are known to produce central nervous system damage. The clinical pictures observed here have been those of generalized encephalopathy and diffuse damage. Organic antimonials, however, have not been known to produce this type of injury. Among the organic tin compounds, the tri-alkyl compounds are especially notorious in producing central nervous system damage with cerebral edema.

Organic Compounds

A variety of organic compounds or classes of organic compounds are known to produce central nervous system injury. Carbon disulfide is one of the more characteristic of these. Whether or not this injury is related to a primary vascular change or injury of nerve cells themselves is yet unknown. The phosphoramides are of interest in that they produce a peripheral nerve involvement and do not penetrate the central nervous system. Butyl Cellosolve has been reported to have produced a prolonged, reversible injury to the central nervous system. This picture has somewhat mimicked multiple sclerosis in some instances. Methyl alcohol and ethyl alcohol have been implicated in chronic intoxications with effects upon the central nervous system. Chronic ethanol poisoning, of course, has produced Korsakoff psychosis and Wernike's encephalopathy. This would seem to be related to thiamine or other vitamin deficiencies occurring with chronic ethanol intake. Methylbromide and methylsulfate have also been found to cause central nervous system damage. Triorthocresyl phosphate produced demyelinization and DFP and Mipafox have also been found to produce similar damage to peripheral nerves and the central nervous system. There are a few cases of intoxication with pyridine of a subacute nature in which vertigo and seventh nerve injury have been described.

I have not included such agents as carbon monoxide, nitriles or cyanides which produce damage via lowering oxygen tension of the central nervous system tissues.

9. *Relationship of Trauma to Neurologic Diseases*

Occupational physicians are confronted occasionally with the question as to whether an occupational injury is the cause of a neurologic disease. This situation arises when a neurologic disease manifests itself for the first time following an injury. In these instances, the symptoms of a neurologic disease may be precipitated or aggravated by an occupational injury. In most instances, we have very few facts to justify the relationship between an injury and a neurologic disease. Neurologic authorities differ widely. Mostly, we have only opinions. People are suggestible; trauma offers an escape from the problems of life; the willingness of many people to sue; and at times, bad management on the part of physicians and lawyers all confuse the picture. The patient is so apt to overexaggerate his troubles in order to make a favorable impression in court. Juries have disregarded medical testimony that no relationship exists between an injury and a neurologic condition and have awarded a settlement on the basis of chronology alone of the events. I was once an expert witness on a case where multiple sclerosis was judged by the jury to have had a direct relationship to the trauma, simply because of the short space of time between injury and onset of symptoms. The following seems to be the state of affairs at present in these neurologic conditions:

1. *General Paresis*

1. Never caused by trauma, although trauma may precipitate or aggravate general paresis. The injury must be to the head and the latent period must not exceed three months. Most of the cases in the literature reported as due to trauma were in the period before the spirochete was known to be the causative agent.

2. *Brain Tumor*

2. Trauma cannot be said to be or not to be the cause of brain tumors, because we do not know the cause of brain tumors. Sarcoma and osteoma have developed at the site of an injury following a blow to the head. Meningiomas have occasionally developed at the site of a blow to the head. Gliomas probably never are caused by a blow to the head. Hemorrhage into a glioma may follow a blow to the head. Any direct relationship must show that the tumor grew at the site of the blow on the head and the latent period must not exceed three months.

3. *Convulsions*

3. Trauma may cause convulsions even if there is no demonstrable clinical brain injury. Convulsions may develop six months to two or more years following the injury, especially if there is scar formation. Focal convulsions (Jacksonian) increase the probability that trauma is the cause. One should rule out the existence of convulsions before the accident. A person with convulsions may have an accident to the head during a convulsion, and the convulsions may become more frequent and intense following the accident because of brain damage. If convulsions develop immediately following a slight blow to the head, one should suspect a history of previous convulsions.

4. *Syryngomyelia*

4. Trauma does not cause syryngomyelia.

5. *Hematomyelia*

5. Trauma does cause hematomyelia which later may cause a syryngomyelic cavity or central gliosis.

6. *Tabes Dorsalis*

6. Trauma does not cause tabes dorsalis, but it might precipitate or aggravate it.

7. *Epidemic Meningitis or Encephalitis*

7. Trauma probably does not cause these conditions, although one may find authorities saying it is possible.

8. *Amyotrophic Lateral Sclerosis*

8. Trauma probably does not cause this condition. The cause is not known.

9. *Multiple Sclerosis*

9. Trauma probably does not cause this condition but the cause is not known so that opinion rules in each individual case. Authorities can be found to substantiate each side of the argument.

10. *Paralysis Agitans*

10. Trauma possibly might cause this condition, but most authorities will not agree.

11. *Cerebral Arteriosclerosis*

11. Trauma may precipitate, aggravate or accelerate a cerebral arteriosclerotic process. The process may have been progressing very slowly before the accident and following the accident the mental deterioration might become accelerated. Also, there may be a rupture of a blood vessel following a head injury in a person who has had symptoms of cerebral arteriolsclerosis. In these instances, authorities have declared that there is a direct relationship between head injury and resulting condition. The apoplexy may occur immediately or after a period of time. The symptoms of cerebral arteriosclerosis have been accelerated by a head blow.

12. *Spinal Cord Tumor*

12. Trauma probably does not cause this condition. Since we do not know the cause of tumors, opinions will rule in each individual case.

13. *Subacute Combined Sclerosis*

13. Trauma does not cause this condition.

14. *Progressive Muscular Atrophy*

14. Trauma does not cause this condition as far as we know. However, since we do not know the cause of this condition, opinions will rule in each individual case.

15. *Progressive Muscular Dystrophy*

15. Trauma does not cause this condition as far as we know. However, since we do not know the cause of this condition, opinions will rule in each individual case.

10. *Neurologic Reminders of Some Muscle Motions and Reflexes*

THE AUTHOR CONSIDERED that a list of certain rather common muscle motions with the corresponding muscles involved, the peripheral nerves which innervated these muscles and the spinal segments of these peripheral nerves might be useful to occupational physicians. I have not included all possible muscle motions because of the limitation of space. In the lists, I have *italicized* the chief muscles and nerves involved and the chief spinal segment involved.

Muscle Motion	Muscles Tested	Peripheral Nerves Tested	Spinal Segments Tested
1. Abduction of arm *toward* the horizontal	*Deltoid*	Axillary	C5-C6
2. Abduction of arm *to* the horizontal	*Deltoid*, supraspinatus, infraspinatus, teres minor, subscapularis	*Axillary* Suprascapular subscapular	C5-C6
3. Elevation of arm over the head	*Deltoid, Supraspinatus*, lateral rotators of scapula, trapezius, serratus anterior	*Axillary (Circumflex) Suprascapular* Subscapular Accessory Long thoracic	C5-C6-C7
4. Elevation (shrugging) of the shoulders	Levator scapulae Upper portion of the trapezius	*Accessory*	C3-C4-C5
5. Pushing test (against a wall)	*Serratus Anterior*	Long thoracic	C5-C6-C7
6. Medial (internal rotation of arm at the shoulder)	*Subscapularis, Teres Major, Deltoid (Anterior Fibers)* latissimus dorsi Pectoralis Major	*Subscapularis Thoracodorsal* Anterior thoracic medial and lateral) Axillary	C-5-C6-C7

*Adapted from *Peripheral Nerve Injuries* by Haymaker and Woodhall, W. B. Saunders, Co., 1945.

7. Lateral rotation (external) of arm at the shoulder	*Infraspinatus* Teres minor Deltoid (post fibers)	*Suprascapular* Axillary	C4-*C5*-C6
8. Forearm flexion at elbow	*Brachialis* *Biceps Brachii* Brachioradialis Pronator teres	*Musculo-* *cutaneous* Radial Medial	C5-C6
9. Forearm extension at elbow	*Triceps Brachii* Anconeus	*Radial*	C7-*C8*-T1
10. Forearm supination	*Biceps Brachii* *Supinator* Brachioradialis	*Musculo-* *cutaneous* *Radial*	C5-*C6*
11. Forearm pronation	*Pronator Teres* Pronator quadratus Flexor carpi radialis Palmaris longus	*Median*	C6-*C7*-C8
12. Wrist dorsal flexion (extension)	*Extensor Carpi* radialis longus *Extensor Carpi* *Radialis Brevis* Extensor carpi ulnaris Extensors of digits	*Radial*	C6-*C7*-C8
13. Palmar flexion of hand at wrist	*Flexor Carpi* *Radialis* *Flexor Carpi* *Ulnaris* Abductor pollicis longus Flexors of fingers sublimus and pro fundus Palmaris longus	*Median* Ulnar Radial	C6-*C7*-C8
14. Adduction of thumb (ulnar)	*Adductor Pollicis* Extensor Pollicis longus Opponens pollicis Flexor pollicis longus Flexor pollicis brevis	*Ulnar* Radial Median	C7-*C8*-T1
15. Abduction of thumb (palmar)	*1st Interossei* (dorsal and palmar)	*Ulnar* Radial	C8-*T1*

Muscle Motion	Muscles Tested	Peripheral Nerves Tested	Spinal Segments Tested
16. Abduction of thumb (radial)	*Abductor Pollicis Longus* *Extensor Pollicis Brevis*	*Radial*	C7-C8
17. Abduction of thumb (palmar)	*Abductor Pollicis Brevis* *Flexor Pollicis Brevis* (both heads) *Abductor Pollicis Longus* *Opponens Pollicis*	*Median* *Ulnar*	C8-T1
17a. Extension of thumb	Extension of Distal Phalanx		
	Extensor Pollicis Longus	Radial	C7-*C8*
	Extension of Proximal Phalanx		
	Extensor Pollicis Brevis Extensor pollicis longus	Radial	*C7*-C8
18. Thumb flexion	*Phalanx Flexion* *Flexor Pollicis Longus* *Proximal Phalanx Flexion* *Flexor Pollicis Longus*	*Median*	C7-C8-*T1*
	Flexor Pollicis Brevis Abductor pollicis brevis Abductor pollicis	*Median* Ulnar	C8-C8-*T1*
19. Opposition of thumb and little finger	*Thumb Opposition* *Opponens Pollicis* Flexor pollicis brevis (deep head) Abductor pollicis brevis	*Median* Ulnar	**C8-*T1***
	Little Finger Opposition *Opponens Digiti Quinti* Flexor digiti quinti	Ulnar	C8-*T1*

20. Finger adduction (excluding thumb)	*Palmar Interossei*	*Ulnar*	C8-T1
21. Abduction of fingers (excluding thumb)	*Dorsal Interossei* Lumbricales Abductor digiti quinti	*Ulnar*	C8-T1
22. Tensing abdominal muscles	*Rectus Abdominis* External oblique Internal oblique	Lower thoracic nerves	T6-L1
23. Flexion of hip	*Iliopsoas* — chiefly	Femoral—chiefly	L1, *L2, L3, L4*
24. Adduction of thigh	*Adductor Magnus* Adductor brevis Adductor longus	*Obturator*— chiefly Sciatic Inferior gluteal— N. to quadratus femoris	*L2, L3,* L4
	Gluteus maximus (lower fibers)	Quadratus femoris	
25. Abduction of thigh and rotation (internal) of leg at hip	*Gluteus Medius* — chiefly	Superior Gluteal	*L4, L5,* S1
26. Rotation (external) of leg at hip	*Gluteus Maximum Obturator Internus* and *Gemelli* — chiefly	*Inferior Gluteal Nerve to Obturator Internus*—chiefly	*L4, L5, S1,* S2
27. Hip extension	*Gluteus Maximus* — chiefly	*Inferior Gluteal* — chiefly	L5, S1, S2
28. Knee extension	*Quadriceps Femoris*	*Femoral*	L2, *L3, L4*
29. Knee flexion	*Biceps Femoris Semitendinosus Semimembranosus*	*Sciatic*	L5, *S1,* S2
30. Foot dorsiflexion	*Tibialis Anterior* — chiefly	*Deep Peroneal*	*L4, L5,* S1
31. Foot plantar flexion	*Gastrocnemius Soleus* — chiefly	*Tibial* — chiefly	*L5, S1, S2,* S3
32. Foot inversion	*Tibialis Posterior Tibialis Anterior* — chiefly	*Posterior Tibial Deep Peroneal*— chiefly	*L4, L5,* S1, S2

Muscle Motion	Muscles Tested	Peripheral Nerves Tested	Spinal Segments Tested
33. Foot eversion	Peroneus Longus Peroneus Brevis — chiefly	Superficial Peroneal Deep Peroneal	L5, S1, S2
34. Dorsiflexion (extension) of toes	Extensor Hallucis Longus — chiefly	Deep Peroneal	L5, S1, S2
35. Plantar flexion toes, great toe	Flexor Hallucis Brevis Flexor Hallucis Longus — chiefly	Posterior Tibial	S1, S2

A list of the deep and superficial reflexes with the resultant reflex action, the mediating nerve and the reflex center is included for ready reference. A few pathologic reflexes are listed with their pathology and significance.

DEEP REFLEXES

Deep Reflex	Reflex Action	Nerve Pathway	Reflex Center
1. Jaw jerk	Raising of jaw by masseter contraction	Trigeminal	pons
2. Pectoral	Adduction and slight internal rotation of humerus	Anterior thoracic	spinal cord
3. Biceps	Flexion of forearm	Musculocutaneous C5, C6	spinal cord
4. Triceps	Extension of forearm	Radial nerve C6, C7	spinal cord
5. Radial	Supination and Flexion at the elbow Occasionally, flexion of wrist and fingers	Radial nerve C7, C8	spinal cord
6. Ulnar	Pronation of hand	Median nerve C8, T1	spinal cord
7. Patellar	Extension of knee Occasionally, ipsi-lateral or crossed adduction of thigh	Femoral nerve L2, L3, L4	spinal cord
8. Suprapatellar	Elevation of patella (part of patellar reflex)	Femoral nerve L2, L3, L4	spinal cord
9. Flexion reflex of leg	Flexion of leg	Sciatic nerve L4, L5, S1, S2	spinal cord

10. Ankle	Ankle plantar flexion	Posterior tibial nerve S1, S2	

SUPERFICIAL REFLEXES

Superficial Reflexes	Reflex Action	Nerve Pathway	Reflex Center
1. Ciliospinal	Pupil dilation	Cervical sympathetic medulla pathway C8, T1	medulla spinal cord
2. Palmar	Flexion of fingers	C8, T1	spinal cord
3. Abdominal — upper	Ipsilateral contraction of abdominal muscles Deviation of linea alba and umbilicus to side stroked	T7, T8	spinal cord
4. Abdominal — middle	Deviation to side stroked	T8, T9	spinal cord
5. Abdominal — lower	Deviation to side stroked	T10, T11	spinal cord
6. Cremasteric	Ipsilateral contraction of cremaster muscle and elevation of testicle	L1, L2	spinal cord
7. Anal	Contraction of external anal sphincter	S5	spinal cord
8. Plantar	Flexion of toes	S1, S2	spinal cord

PATHOLOGIC REFLEXES

Pathologic Reflex	Reflex Action	Pathologic Significance
1. *Babinski toe sign* (stroking upward and inward outer side of sole of foot)	Fanning and plantar flexion of smaller toes Dorsiflexion (extension) of big toe	1. Pyramidal tract disease 2. Narcosis 3. General coma 4. Postconvulsive state
2. *Flexion reflex of legs* (Stroking surface of feet, leg or thigh or passive bending of toes)	Mass flexion withdrawal reflex	1. Pyramidal tract disease
3. *Grasp reflex* (Stroking palm and fingers)	Closure of hand on stimulating object	Frontal lobe lesions

Pathologic Reflex	Reflex Action	Pathologic Significance
4. *Mass reflex*	Flexion reflex of legs Contraction of abdominal wall Automatic evacuation of bladder Sweating of skin below level of lesion	Complete interruption or severe injury of spinal cord
5. *Oculocardiac reflex* Normally, pressure on eyeballs produces slowing of pulse	In *sympathicotonics* reflex is diminished or absent In *vagotonics* it is exaggerated	Abolished often in tabes exaggerated in exophthalmic goiter

NEUROLOGIC ILLUSTRATIONS OF SPINAL SEGMENTS, PERIPHERAL NERVES AND MUSCLE INNERVATIONS

The author has selected the following diagrams and tables which he hopes will aid the occupational physician in understanding the innervation of skin and muscles by spinal segments and the distribution of the peripheral nerves. These were reproduced from the book, *Peripheral Nerve Injuries*, by Haymaker and Woodhall.

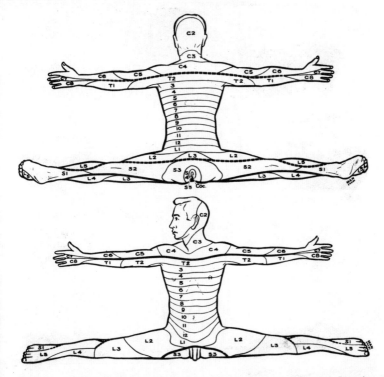

Fig. 1—*Diagram to Illustrate the Position of Ventral* (in Solid Lines) *and Dorsal* (in Broken Lines) *Axial Lines.* The axial lines of the upper limb extend down the middle of the corresponding surfaces. In the lower limb, the ventral axial line starts in the region of the pubis and winds round the inner side of the thigh to gain the back of the thigh and subsequently the calf; the dorsal line, after crossing the upper part of the buttock, pursues a course down the more lateral part of the leg to the region of the ankle. The dermatomic pattern is after Foerster in Haymaker and Woodhall: Peripheral Nerve Injuries. Philadelphia, W. B. Saunders Co., 1945.)

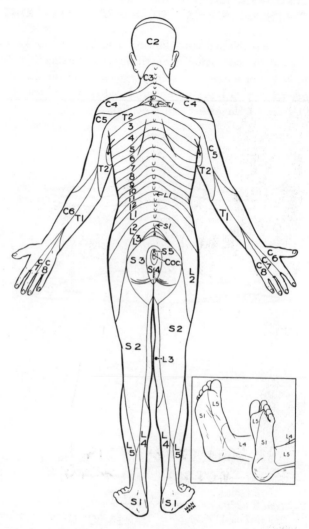

Fig. 2.—*The Dermatomes from the Posterior View.* Note the absence of cutaneous innervation by the first cervical segment. Arrows in the axillary regions indicate the lateral extent of dermatome T3; those in the region of the vertebral column point to the first thoracic, the first lumbar and the first sacral spinous processes (After Foerster in Haymaker and Woodhall: Peripheral Nerve Injuries. Philadelphia, W. B. Saunders Co., 1945.)

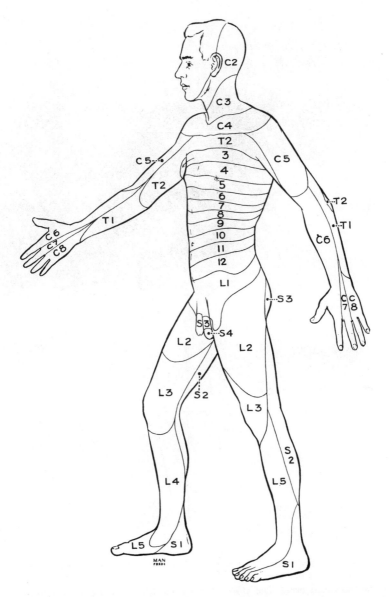

Fig. 3.—*A Side View of the Dermatomes.* (After Foerster in Haymaker and Woodhall: Peripheral Nerve Injuries. Philadelphia, W. B. Saunders Co., 1945.)

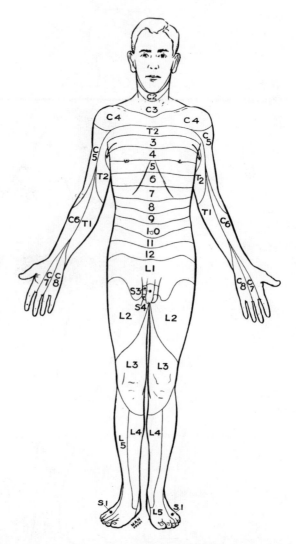

FIG. 4.—*The Segmental Innervation of the Skin from the Anterior Aspect.*
The uppermost dermatome adjoins the cutaneous field of the mandibular division
of the trigeminal nerve. The arrows indicate the lateral extensions of dermatome
T3. (After Foerster in Haymaker and Woodhall: Peripheral Nerve Injuries. Philadelphia, W. B. Saunders Co., 1945.)

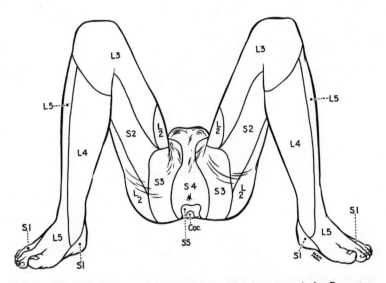

Fig. 5—*Perineal View of the Body Showing the Location of the Dermatomes.*
From Haymaker and Woodhall: Peripheral Nerve Injuries. Philadelphia, W. B.
Saunders Co., 1945.

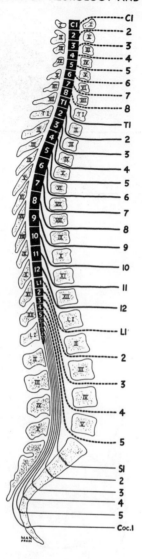

FIG. 6—*The Alignment of Spinal Segments with Vertebrae.* The bodies and spinous processes of the vertebrae are indicated by Roman numerals, the spinal segments and their respective nerves by Arabic. It will be noted that the cervical nerves take exit through intervertebral foramina *above* their respective vertebral bodies and that the other nerves issue *below* these bodies. From Haymaker and Woodhall: Peripheral Nerve Injuries. Philadelphia, W. B. Saunders Co., 1945.

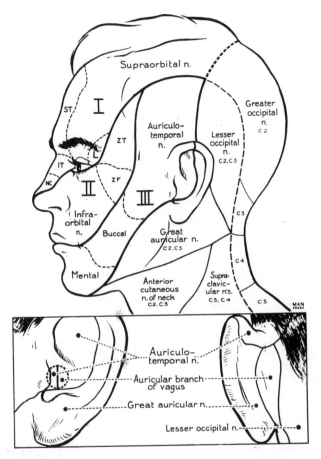

Fig. 7.—*Diagram of the Cutaneous Fields of the Head and Upper Part of the Neck.* The three divisions of the trigeminal nerve (I, ophthalmic; II, maxillary; III, mandibular) are indicated by heavy lines, and their respective subdivisions by light broken lines. The conjunctivae are innervated by the ophthalmic division. Abbreviations refer to the following nerves: B, buccal; IT, infratrochlear; L, lacrymal; NC, external nasal branch of the nasociliary; ST, supratrochlear; ZF, zygomaticofacial; ZT, zygomaticotemporal. The lateral and superior boundaries of the posterior primary rami are indicated by broken lines. The inset shows trigeminal and vagal cutaneous fields of the region of the external ear and the external auditory meatus. From Haymaker and Woodhall: Peripheral Nerve Injuries. Philadelphia, W. B. Saunders Co., 1945.

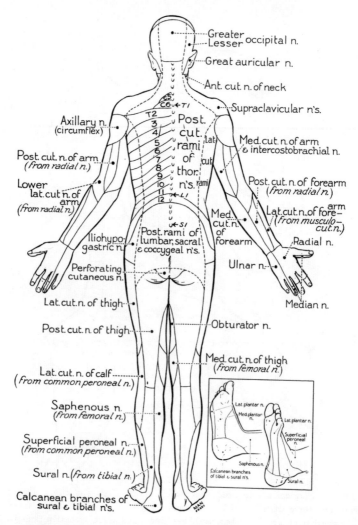

FIG. 8.—*The Cutaneous Fields of Peripheral Nerves from the Posterior Aspect.*
The boundaries of cutaneous supply of the posterior primary rami are indicated by
broken lines. The designation, *Post. cut. rami of thor. n's.*, refers to the cutaneous
branches of the posterior primary rami; *Lat. cut. rami* indicates the distribution
from the lateral branches of the anterior primary rami. For purposes of orientation
the spinous processes of the first thoracic (T1), the first number (L1) and the
first sacral (S1) vertebrae are indicated by arrows. From Haymaker and Woodhall:
Peripheral Nerve Injuries. Philadelphia. W. B. Saunders Co., 1945.

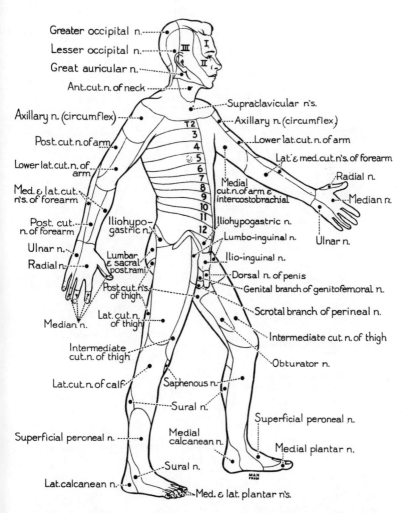

Greater occipital n.
Lesser occipital n.
Great auricular n.
Ant. cut. n. of neck
Axillary n. (circumflex)
Post. cut. n. of arm
Lower lat. cut. n. of arm
Med. & lat. cut. n's. of forearm
Post. cut. n. of forearm
Ulnar n.
Radial n.
Iliohypogastric n.
Lumbar & sacral post. rami
Post. cut. n's. of thigh
Lat. cut. n. of thigh
Median n.
Intermediate cut. n. of thigh
Lat. cut. n. of calf
Superficial peroneal n.
Lat. calcanean n.

Supraclavicular n's.
Axillary n. (circumflex)
Lower lat. cut. n. of arm
Lat. & med. cut. n's. of forearm
Radial n.
Median n.
Medial cut. n. of arm & intercostobrachial
Iliohypogastric n.
Ulnar n.
Lumbo-inguinal n.
Ilio-inguinal n.
Dorsal n. of penis
Genital branch of genitofemoral n.
Scrotal branch of perineal n.
Intermediate cut. n. of thigh
Obturator n.
Saphenous n.
Sural n.
Superficial peroneal n.
Medial plantar n.
Medial calcanean n.
Sural n.
Med. & lat. plantar n's.

I, II, III, T2, 3, 4, 5, 6, 7, 8, 9, 10, 11, 12

MANFRED

FIG. 9.—*Side View of the Cutaneous Fields of Peripheral Nerves.* The face and anterior half of the head are innervated by the three divisions of the trigeminal: I, ophthalmic; II, maxillary; III, mandibular. The fields of the intercostal nerves are indicated by numerals. The unlabeled cutaneous field between great and second toe is supplied by the deep peroneal nerve. From Haymaker and Woodhall: Peripheral Nerve Injuries. Philadelphia, W. B. Saunders Co., 1945.

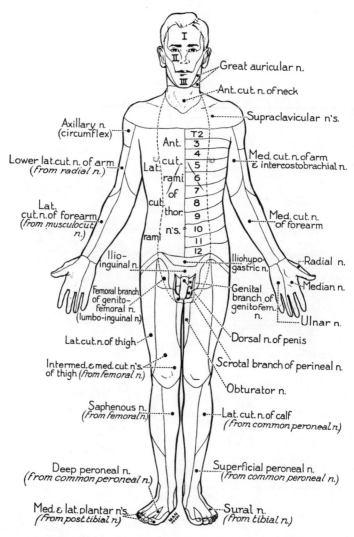

FIG. 10.—*The Cutaneous Fields of Peripheral Nerves from the Anterior Aspect.*
The numbers on the left side of the trunk refer to the intercostal nerves. On the
right side are shown the cutaneous fields of the lateral and medial branches of
the anterior primary rami. The asterisk just beneath the scrotum is in the field
of the posterior cutaneous nerve of the thigh. From Haymaker and Woodhall:
Peripheral Nerve Injuries. Philadelphia, W. B. Saunders Co., 1945.

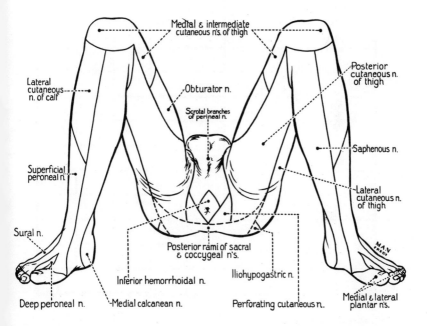

FIG. 11.—*Perineal View of the Cutaneous Fields of Peripheral Nerves.* From Haymaker and Woodhall: Peripheral Nerve Injuries. Philadelphia, W. B. Saunders Co., 1945.

TABLE 1.—*Segmental Innervation of Muscles of the Neck, Shoulder and Upper Arm*

Muscle	SPINAL SEGMENTS								
	C1	C2	C3	C4	C5	C6	C7	C8	T1
Sternomastoid*	▮	▮	▮	▮					
Trapezius*		▮	▮	▮					
Levator scapulae			▮	▮	▮				
Teres minor				▮	▮				
Supraspinatus				▮	▮	▮			
Rhomboids				▮	▮				
Infraspinatus				▮	▮	▮			
Deltoid					▮	▮			
Teres major					▮	▮	▮		
Biceps					▮	▮			
Brachialis					▮	▮			
Serratus anterior					▮	▮	▮		
Subscapularis					▮	▮	▮	▮	
Pectoralis major					▮	▮	▮	▮	▮
Pectoralis minor						▮	▮	▮	▮
Coraco-brachialis						▮	▮		
Latissimus dorsi						▮	▮	▮	
Anconeus							▮	▮	
Triceps							▮	▮	▮

The asterisks indicate a supply also from the accessory nerve. A line bisecting a segment indicates that the muscle receives minor innervation from that segment.

Modified after Bing in Haymaker and Woodhall: Peripheral Nerve Injuries. Philadelphia, W. B. Saunders Co., 1945.

TABLE 2.—*Segmental Innervation of Muscles of the Forearm and Hand*

SPINAL SEGMENTS				
C5	C6	C7	C8	T1
Brachioradialis				
Supinator				
	Pronator teres			
	Ext. carpi radial. longus & brevis			
	Flexor carpi ulnaris			
	Flexor carpi radialis			
		Ext. digitorum		
		Ext. carpi ulnaris		
		Ext. indicis		
		Ext. digiti 5		
		Ext. pollic. longus		
		Ext. pollic. brevis		
		Abductor pollicis longus		
		Palmaris longus		
		Pronator quadratus		
		Flexor digitorum sublimis		
		Flexor digitorum profundus		
		Flexor pollicis longus		
			Opponens pollicis	
			Abduct. pollic. brevis	
			Flexor pollicis brevis	
			Palmaris brevis	
			Adductor pollicis	
			Flexor digiti 5	
			Abductor digiti 5	
			Opponens digiti 5	
			Interossei	
		Lumbricals		

A line bisecting a segment indicates that the muscle receives minor innervation from that segment.

Modified after Bing in Haymaker and Woodhall: Peripheral Nerve Injuries. Philadelphia, W. B. Saunders Co., 1945.

TABLE 3.—*Segmental Innervation of Muscles of the Hip and Thigh*

Muscle	L1	L2	L3	L4	L5	S1	S2
SPINAL SEGMENTS							
Iliopsoas	X	X	X	X			
Gracilis		X	X	X			
Sartorius		X	X	X			
Pectineus		X	X	X			
Adductor longus		X	X	X			
Adductor brevis		X	X	X			
Adductor minimus		X	X	X			
Quadratus femoris		X	X	X	X		
Adductor magnus		X	X	X	X		
Obturator externus			X	X	X		
Tensor fasciae latae				X	X	X	
Gluteus medius				X	X	X	
Gluteus minimus				X	X	X	
Quadriceps femoris				X	X	X	X
Gemelli				X	X	X	X
Semitendinosus				X	X	X	X
Semimembranosus				X	X	X	X
Piriformis					X	X	X
Obturator internus					X	X	X
Biceps femoris					X	X	X
Gluteus maximus					X	X	X

A line bisecting a segment indicates that the muscle receives minor innervation from that segment.

Modified after Bing in Haymaker and Woodhall: Peripheral Nerve Injuries. Philadelphia, W. B. Saunders Co., 1945.

TABLE 4.—*Segmental Innervation of Muscles of the Leg and Foot*

Muscle	SPINAL SEGMENTS			
	L4	L5	S1	S2
Tibialis anterior	X	X		
Popliteus	X	X	X	
Plantaris	X	X	X	
Peroneus tertius	X	X	X	
Extensor digitorum longus	X	X	X	X
Abductor hallucis		X	X	
Flexor digitorum brevis		X	X	
Flexor hallucis brevis		X	X	
Extensor hallucis brevis		X	X	
Flexor digitorum longus		X	X	X
Peroneus longus		X	X	X
Peroneus brevis		X	X	X
Tibialis posterior		X	X	
Flexor hallucis longus		X	X	
Extensor hallucis longus		X	X	
Soleus		X	X	
Gastrocnemius			X	X
Extensor digitorum brevis			X	X
Flexor digitorum accessorius			X	X
Adductor hallucis			X	X
Abductor digiti quinti			X	X
Flexor digiti quinti brevis			X	X
Interossei			X	X
Lumbricals		X	X	

A line bisecting a segment indicates that the muscle receives minor innervation from that segment.

Modified after Bing in Haymaker and Woodhall: Peripheral Nerve Injujries. Philadelphia, W. B. Saunders Co., 1945.

11. *Psychiatry at the Work Place (Occupational Psychiatry)*

OCCUPATIONAL PHYSICIANS usually see a cross-section of the community citizenry in their daily work. The usual illnesses will be seen, togther with those ailments peculiar to the occupational setting. They will see physical illnesses with emotional overtones and emotional illnesses by themselves. Emotional and mental illnesses are very common in our daily life and they should be understood by physicians. The following are some facts apropos to this situation in any work place, viz:

1. Emotional illnesses cause more absenteeism than all other illnesses save the common cold.

2. 25 per cent of workers have personality disorders showing up in: 1. Absenteeism. 2. Alcoholism. 3. Accidents. 4. Illness. 5. Job dissatisfaction. 6. Trouble with co-workers and supervisors.

3. 60 to 80 per cent of dismissals are due to social incompetence (1920) — today people say it is 90 per cent. 20 to 40 per cent of dismissals are due to technical incompetence (1920) — today people say it is 10 per cent.

4. 60 to 70 per cent of medical complaints which occupational workers bring to the dispensary are emotional in origin. Many physical diseases have many emotional overtones which delay the recovery from the physical illness.

5. Mental illness and emotional attitudes are communicable. This affects the emotional climate of office, shops and departments, and even companies.

6. The occupational physician should be able to detect emotional illnesses early and, with minor psychotherapy, help the employee to recover and to prevent a major breakdown.

7. Mental patients occupy more than 50 per cent of the total hospital beds in the U.S.

8. Many states allot 40 to 60 per cent of their budgets to the care of the mentally ill.

9. The emotional climate and the emotional attitude of workers of a department are influenced by the health and attitudes of the department leader.

10. Good mental health of all of the employees at any level is important because it will foster the following, viz:

1. Increase production. 2. Increase better attitudes. 3. Increase job satisfaction. 4. Decrease absenteeism. 5. Decrease accidents. 6. Decrease alcoholism.

11. Employees want certain things out of their jobs — does the occupational physician know these wants? If the employee does not get these things he may develop emotional symptoms and unhealthy attitudes. These usually have been stated as follows, viz:

1. Job security. 2. Job satisfaction. 3. Job recognition. 4. Job promotion. Job salary.

Salary is usually way down on the list and this is the only tangible item on the list — all the others are intangible items — difficult to measure. Tredgold states the following reasons as to why people work, viz:

"1. A search for material security. 2. Personal responsibility. 3. A desire to conform to type. 4. The desire for the approval of the group 5. The desire for preeminence. 6. Pride in skill. 7. A sense of order. 8. Acquisitiveness. 9. A compelling conscientiousness."

12. Every company has a personality — we call it the corporate personality — and the occupational physician should be aware of this as he then will be better able to understand some of the complaints, the attitudes and the behavior of his employees whom he sees in the Medical Department. Each company attracts certain types of personalities to it.

13. Techniques of interviewing, counselling and minor psychotherapy should be mastered by occupational physicians.

14. Group dynamics are important in the understanding of employees' illnesses, as many employees will develop emotional illnesses because of group forces that are operating on them.

15. Leadership based on an interest in people, and an understanding of people, their needs and desires in life, and at the work place, together with mature and sound judgement in relationship to policy making will produce a sound, effective and healthy climate for people who work. This is preventive mental health. The education of supervision at any level in any company is necessary if they are to understand people and to manage people with concern, with enlightenment, and with fairness.

16. Emotional factors will arise many times in compensation injuries. The occupational physician should know the facts of this situation.

17. "A neurosis always has psychological meaning," declare Bond, Flumerfelt and Bidder.[2] They continue:

... its general significance is that it is a pathologic attempt on the part of the patient to maintain a harmonious adjustment within himself among the demands of instinct, of conscience, and of reality. It is the patient's way of taking half a loaf of satisfaction rather than none. It is an error to assume, however, that whatever obvious gain the patient derives from his neurosis is the cause of it. Such is never the case. In fact, the patient himself is seldom aware of the real cause. Furthermore, each separate neurotic symptom has a specific meaning, part of which meaning may be obvious to an outsider, but not to the patient.

18. The management of the neurotic, the psychopath and the psychotic employee at the work place should be familiar to the occupational physician.

19. The occupational physician may be interested in what Ling says in his book Mental Health and Human Relations in Industry about human problems in industry, viz:

Since World War I there has been a rapidly developing interest in the human problems of industry. Why do people work? And why do they strike? Why is absenteeism so high in one industry and low in another? Why do people want to put their children into one trade and make equal efforts to keep them away from another? These are not just recondite questions but matters relevant to this time and age in all industrialized countries. Again, in all countries, one is struck by the evident happiness of many people in their hard-working leisure and their evident dissatisfaction during their working day.

One example will suffice. In the countryside around any big city in England early on a Sunday morning one can see young men pedalling bicycles in amateur long-distance races with an enthusiasm that has to be seen to be believed. Sweat drips from their brows, their girl-friends have turned out to support them, other amateurs measure the time with stop watches and the bicyclists themselves appear keen and alive. These same people at their jobs in the factory look, feel and behave differently. They will often appear bored, irritated, frustrated and tense, probably grumbling about the management and perhaps watching the clock until they can leave. Some will be political extremists, others just the rather unhappy people who are to be found in every industrial community.

In the first named situation, they earn no money for their hard work on their bicycles but appear happy and cooperative. In the second, they draw good wages at the end of the week but are often unhappy in the process. In the first named situation, everyone will turn up if they can possibly manage it; in the factory, escape into strikes, absenteeism, illness and psychosomatic breakdown is unduly common. Why the great difference? What is it that makes the first situation so vital and the second so unsatisfying? The answers are not simple but are the keys to industrial mental health and to a high level of productivity in all industrialized countries.

REFERENCES

1. Tredgold, R. F.: Human Relations in Modern Industry. New York, International Universities Press, Inc., 1949.
2. Bond, D. D., Flumerfelt, J. M., Bidder, T. G.: Psychiatry. In Cecil, R. L. and Conn, H. F., Eds.: The Specialties in General Practice, ed. 2. Philadelphia and London, Chapt. 14. W. B. Saunders Co., 1957.
3. Ling, T. M.: Mental Health and Human Relations in Industry. London. H. K. Lewis & Co. Ltd., 1954.

12.   *Psychiatric History Reminders*

THE OCCUPATIONAL PHYSICIAN who has an interest in the total health of his employees will want to know how to detect the presence or absence of emotional or/and environmental factors in the illness of the employee, how to evaluate these factors, how to handle them within the occupational setting, and when and to whom to refer those employees who need to be referred for further therapy.

Occupational physicians have become more knowledgeable about these emotional, personality and environmental factors in recent years, because they have been convinced that these factors play a tremendously important role, not only in the total life of the employee, but also specifically in his work life, in the health and effectiveness of the company, and also in the off-the-job life of the employee. Occupational physicians have been attending special courses in occupational psychiatry which have been given at various medical and psychiatric teaching centers in the U. S. during the past few years for the specific purpose of orienting them in this field.

This section of the monograph will attempt to set down some guiding reminders on the subject for those who are interested. Those readers who may have a deeper interest in psychiatry are referred to standard textbooks of psychiatry and allied subjects.

"Acceptance" of psychiatric findings in medicine has been greatly aided by the work of psychologists, Pavlov, Cannon, Harold G. Wolff and many others, who have made concrete for the physician the neural and humoral pathways over which emotional discharges may flow to influence function and structure in various bodily parts. At the same time, the discovery of the benefits of shock therapy (von Meduna, Sakel, Cerletti and Bini) has stimulated much interest in the organic influence upon the mental process in the psychoses. To date, however, this later trend of investigation has failed to add to our present knowledge of the psychological processes.

Since the increased recognition of the emotional influence in dysfunction, physicians have been less baffled by many syndromes. Although there are no reliable over-all statistics to support the following claim, many outstanding internists have estimated that as many as 50 to 60 per cent of the patients whom they see suffer primarily from emotional disturbances. This observation has tended to cut down the number of fruitless laboratory examinations and to discourage a former tendency to blame some minor physical defect for many different kinds of symptoms. Fortunately, too, this observation has decreased the tendency to overtreat many illnesses or to lay undue emphasis on relatively unimportant findings."[1]

The occupational physician who is unsure of his knowledge about the field of emotional disorders because he has had no formal training in it, can be assurred that he can be an effective therapist if he would but have the following qualifications, viz.:

1. A *belief* that *emotions, feeling, attitudes, ideas* and *environment* can affect the health of the employee by causing physical reactions and symptoms.

2. An ever-present attitude during the history taking and examination that *there may always be emotional and environmental factors present.*

3. *A belief that behavior has meaning* and *one should always look for that meaning.*

4. Patience and a determination to be an interested and sympathetic listener while the employee verbalizes his troubles.

5. A personality that assures the employee that the physician is sympathetic, warm, nonthreatening, nonjudicial and interested in the employee.

6. A desire to learn more about this area of medicine.

The following points should be considered relative to psychiatric history taking in an occupational setting:

1. Most of the people whom one sees in an occupational setting will be troubled people, i.e., people who are average persons with no symptoms of mental illness but who are having trouble with the every-day problems of living and develop physical and emotional symptoms.

2. Patience has its rewards — one must not get discouraged after a few interviews if one does not put one's finger on the personality or environmental factors causing the symptoms. One may never find out, but the patient gets better anyway. "Uncovering" therapy (revealing deep, unconscious psychological mechanisms) is seldom applicable to the occupational setting.

3. Just listening may allow the patient to ventilate sufficiently so that he may function again at an effective level for him, without symptoms.

4. During a recitation of symptoms, the physician may gather significant data if he but listens and tries to correlate symptomatology and dates of onset with events in the patient's life.

5. If the physician feels that there are emotional factors involved and he cannot spend any more time that day with the employee, he should make another appointment to spend more time with his investigation. These so-called neurotic patients can take up an inordinate amount of the physician's time in repeated visits over many months if all the physician does is to treat symptoms and does not carry out some pertinent questioning about the individual, his life, attitudes, emotions and goals in life. A few interviews of 30 minutes each can solve many problems and yet the total time may be less than when the patient sees the physician repeatedly during which visits the doctor only spends a few minutes each time with the patient. Doctors have said that they cannot take time from their busy practices in order to sit down and spend 30 minutes with a neurotic patient. However, if more time is spent in a few interviews, more can be accomplished, and the patient won't be returning so often to the Medical Department.

6. Employees are known by physicians for years, and this allows the physicians to really get to know them, their families, their hopes, their goals in life, their job problems. Also, the physician has available the knowledge of these same employees from their foremen and from the Personnel Department, from the nurses, etc. A body of data through the years is built up about each employee, and this is really social data which can be invaluable in treating the employee.

7. Likewise, through many contacts with the physician over the years, the employee builds up confidence in the physician and the nurses, if, by their practices and their warm friendly and interested personalities they have instilled in the employee the confidence which is necessary for the development of a healthy climate in the Medical Department.

8. The personality of the physician is a potent and an important aspect of the patient-physician relationship, especially when dealing with an emotional problem. One has heard patients say, "Why, the minute the doctor walked into the room, I felt better." This is another tool which the physician can develop and exploit in his ferreting out of the causes of an employee's illness.

Psychiatric history-taking begins when the patient begins to recite his complaints about how he feels, his symptoms, etc.

History-taking Reminders

1. Let the patient tell his story uninterruptedly. One may fill in the gaps later.

2. Put the patient at ease — the physician should give the patient the impression that there is plenty of time for the patient to tell the story.

3. Observe the patient closely during the recitation of the story — his reactions, the facial expressions, emotional reactions, his behavior, whether

restlessness is present or not, tone of voice (with feeling or not), flow of words or slowing of speech. (These are actually part of the psychiatric examination, but they should be registered in the physician's mind during the history-taking and the physical examination, as they are part of the psychologic survey.)

4. When the patient has finished the story, the physician should then begin to fill in the gaps in the history, viz.: when did the symptoms begin, how did it begin, has he ever had it before, with what is it associated in his life, etc. The physician should make the usual system survey from head to toe, covering past illnesses, accidents, injuries, fractures, operations, hospitalizations, compensation experiences, etc. The usual medical and physical history can be woven into this history-taking. The family history may be significant, as other members of the family may have had symptoms similar to the patient's symptoms (identification syndrome).

5. Depending on the time the physician can give to the patient on the first visit, he will determine the extent of his questioning before he examines the patient. At times, the physician will not have the time to do a complete physical examination, but he should always examine that part of the patient's body about which he is complaining. This will give the patient the impression that the physician is interested.

6. During the examination, the doctor often picks up other tidbits of history which are important. (The patient may digress and talk of completely extraneous topics during the history-taking and the physical examination. These should be registered in the physician's mind, or mentioned at the time with such questions as "I wonder why you talked about that — does it bother you?")

7. After the examination the patient should be allowed a few moments to talk, as he might have thought of other things to talk about from being stimulated by the physician's interest in him, his complaints, his body and his health.

8. *Further history* to be taken about the patient's complaints, his personal, cultural and social background, might follow this outline, viz.:

(1) Job, job reactions, and feelings about the job.

(2) Occupational history.

(3) Birth and early development.

(4) School history.

(5) Early family life, including impressions of parents, brothers, sisters.

(6) Marital history.

(7) Religious history.

(8) Sex history.

(9) Miscellaneous personal factors that the examiner may be curious about.

9. If the physician, after a thorough physical examination and laboratory

procedures, believes that there is no organic disease, he then may tell the patient exactly that. He then may say, "Although I do not find anything physical to cause your complaints, there may be some emotional or nervous factors that may cause your trouble, and maybe we might talk about some of these things. Tell me, how is your job going these days?" This leads directly into the work area. Since this area of investigation is not as loaded emotionally for the patient as some other areas of investigation may be, he will soon be at ease and will not feel that he is threatened. This questioning may consume a few interviews, but it is always revealing and helpful.

10. *Feelings and job reactions: These are suggested questions to start with.* Others will be thought of as the questioning continues.

(1) How is the job coming along?

(2) Do you like what you are doing?

(3) What kind of a supervisor do you have?

(4) How do you get along with the people you work with?

(5) What do you do on your job? (The physician should visit the work area of the patient to see what the operation is.)

(6) Do you get satisfaction from your job?

(7) When you were in school, what did you want to do when you grew up?

(8) Are you on an hourly basis for your salary, or are you on the incentive system?

(9) Have you thought much about promotion? Where do you want to go in the company?

These questions will open up the subject of his present job and may contribute much data to the cause of his emotional upset. Many times the emotional disorder is caused by feelings and ideas from several areas of the employee's life.

11. *Occupational history*

(1) Make a list of the various jobs the employee has had in his life, why he took them, and why he left them (personal and job stability).

(2) How did you get along with your supervisors and your colleagues on these other jobs? (Ability to take orders, work with others, social flexibility.)

(3) Were you ever fired from a job? Why? (Can't conform, can't take orders, immaturity.)

(4) Did you ever resign from a job? Why? ·(Immaturity, restlessness, job dissatisfaction.)

(5) What kind of a job has your wife wanted you to have? Is she satisfied with your job now? (Proud wife, social climbing tendencies of wife.)

12. *Birth and early development*

(1) Where were you born? How long did you live in that city? (Family travels.)

(2) What cities did you live in? Which one did you like best? Least? Why?

(3) Did you mind moving around? (Ability to mix easily or with difficulty in adjusting to new surroundings and people.)

(4) How did you get along with your playmates in the cities in which you lived? (Ability to adjust socially.)

(5) Do you remember any particular events in your early life that made a deep impression on you? (Traumatic and pleasant experiences.)

13. *School history*

(1) What school did you last attend? (Avoid asking the question, "How far did you go in school?" as this tends to be traumatic and embarrasses the person.)

(2) Did you graduate?

(3) Why did you leave school? (Supplies data as to motivation for learning, family stresses on children to help support the family, and at times, on ability to learn and on level of intelligence.)

(4) Did you repeat any grades?

(5) Did you like to study?

(6) How did you get along with your schoolmates? (Sociability, adjustability.)

(7) How did you get along with your teachers? (Ability to get along with elders, with those in authority, etc.)

14. *Early family life*

(1) What kind of a family did you have? (Personalities surrounding employee.)

(2) What kind of family life did you have? (Pleasant, rigid, flexible, happy, unhappy, responsible parents, alcoholic parents, strict.)

(3) Tell me, what kind of a person was your Father? Mother?

(4) Did you work and play as a family group? Picnics? Travel? Sports activities? Projects around the house? (An index as to structure of family and interest of parents in the family as a whole.)

(5) Did your parents show their love to you?

(6) Was there a favorite child in the family?

(7) Was there much quarreling between your parents?

(8) Did you have chores to do in the house?

(9) How did you get along with your brothers and sisters? Were you a leader or a follower? (Aggressiveness and submissiveness.)

(10) What kind of a neighborhood did you live in?

(11) What kind of schooling did your father have?

(12) Did your mother work outside the home?

(13) What occupation did your father have? Did he change jobs often? (Stability of father.)

(14) Was there much sickness in your family?

15. *Marital history*

(1) When did you marry?

(2) How has your marriage been going?

(3) How long were you engaged? How long did you know your husband (wife) before marriage?

(4) Does your husband (wife) work outside the home? Where?

(5) Do you and your husband (wife) talk with each other about the family problems? (Surprisingly, communications between husband and wife are limited in many instances and this fact leads to much difficulty within the family.)

(6) What are your pet peeves about your mate? And vice-versa?

(7) Do you and your mate go out together occasionally by yourselves?

(8) Do you have disagreements about money?

(9) Does anyone else live with you, other than your family?

16. *Religious history*

(1) Do you belong to a church? Does your mate?

(2) Do you attend a church regularly? Your mate?

(3) Do the children attend Sunday School? What religious instruction do they get?

(4) How do you feel about religion?

(5) Do you have any conflicts with yourself or your wife about religion.

(6) Did you have religious instruction as you were growing up?

17. *Sex history*

(1) Did you have any sex instruction from your parents?

(2) What attitude did you have towards sex as you were growing up?

(3) What conflicts did you have about sex when you were younger?

(4) (If married) Is your sex life satisfactory now? If not, why not?

18. *Miscellaneous items*

(1) Pertinent items that may have aroused the curiosity of the physician as the above questioning proceeded.

REFERENCES

1. Bond, D. D.; Flumerfelt, J. M.; Bidder, T. G.; Cecil, R. L., and Conn, H. F.: Eds.: Psychiatry. The Specialties in General Practice. Philadelphia and London, W. B. Saunders Company, 1957.

13. *Psychiatric Examination Reminders*

OCCUPATIONAL PHYSICIANS should have some idea as to how to cover certain areas of psychologic functioning so that a more complete understanding of the employee is obtained. At times, a proper diagnosis and a method of procedure can be decided upon from the data supplied by the patient as he tells his story of his troubles. At other times, more data are necessary, and the physician should have an outline in mind so that he can assess the psychological functionings. Every patient should be assured that what he tells the occupational physician is confidential and will not be divulged to anybody unless the patient assents. Strict confidentiality on the part of the occupational physician develops confidence by the employees in the medical department, which, in turn, over the years, will be better able to serve the total health needs of the work force at any level. It is assumed, of course, that prior to the psychiatric examination, a general medical history has been taken and physical and neurologic examinations will have been made.

There is no secret known only to psychiatrists as to how to conduct a psychiatric examination. By using a few techniques that psychiatrists have devised, by alert observation and a lot of common sense, the interested occupational physician can conduct an adequate psychiatric examination for his purposes. Because of their training and clinical experience, psychiatrists may evaluate the results of a psychiatric examination differently, but the interested occupational physician can come to a fairly adequate conclusion so that he will be in a position to decide what to do.

The following areas should be covered, viz.:

1. General behavior
2. Thought processes
3. Stream of thought
4. Emotional reaction (Affect)
5. General knowledge
6. Memory and orientation
7. General intelligence
8. Insight and judgment

General Behavior

The examiner should observe the patient closely as the interview progresses and the examination proceeds. He should watch the type of facial expression, the degree of activity, and whether there is a dis-harmony between the actions, the thinking and the emotional expres-sions of the patient. He should note the dress and grooming of the patient and the general attitude toward the doctor and the general situ-ation. Is the activity rigid and stereotyped? Easy or constrained? Is agitation present? Are there any particular gestures, face-picking or finger-picking, or nail-biting? Is the patient restless, or does he sit quietly and stare at the floor or into space?

It is always wise at some point in the evaluation of the patient to question the relatives, if this is possible. Many times the relatives have noticed a change in the patient early in the patient's illness and may suspect that something is not right. In the occupational setting, relatives usually are not there, but a phone call from the doctor may reveal some interesting and important information. Often the relatives will call the doctor before the patient is seen to advise the doctor of changes in behavior, thinking and emotions.

In the following chart, I have made a few possible interpretations of various types of behavior, viz:

General Behavior	Interpretations
1. Overactivity (on the go, can't sit still)	1. Hypomanic or a manic reaction, anxiety reaction
2. Underactivity (sits still, moves slowly and infrequently)	2. Depression, situational (extern-ally caused) or psychotic (internally caused) schizophrenic reactions, es-pecially the catatonic type — a shy, meek, mild, passive personality — mentally retarded
3. Restlessness (shifting position in the chair constantly, pacing floor, etc.)	3. Anxiety reaction, agitated depres-sion
4. Odd behavior (strange acts in disharmony with ideation and emotional expression, seemingly purposeless)	4. Schizoid personality, odd person-ality, confusional state secondary to a hypoglycemic or convulsive epi-sode
5. Chain smoking, nail biting	5. Anxiety reaction, phobic reaction, agitated depression, obsessive com-pulsive reaction
6. Confusion, mixed up, disoriented	6. Schizophrenic reaction (younger patients) senile and presenile re-actions (older patients) brain tumor, brain abscess (if head injury his-

General Behavior	Interpretations
	tory) acute psychotic depression, postconvulsive confusional reaction, toxic and metabolic reactions as hypoglycemia, petit mal episode, immature personality
7. Angriness, argumentativeness	7. Paranoid reaction, anger from justifiable reasons, senile and presenile reactions, immature personality with active projection mechanism, querulous, contentious personality
8. Staring into space	8. Schizoid personality, depression, schizophrenia, petit mal at time of seizure
9. Feeling compelled to do things in a certain way, to check and recheck acts, believing that something will happen if a certain act is not done at a certain time or/and in a certain way.	9. Obsessive compulsive reaction — usually stereotypy of certain schizophrenic states
10. "Things have got to be perfect, Doctor."	10. Obsessive compulsive reaction
11. Stereotypy of attitude, gestures, motions, acts, and of speech	11. Obsessive compulsive reaction
12. Change in usual behavior	12. Schizophrenic states, depressive reactions

Thought Processes

The physician will have observed the flow of speech in his conversation with the patient. Does he talk easily or with difficulty? Does there seem to be pressure behind his speech? Is he fumbling for words? Is he slowed up in his thinking? The occupational physician may have the advantage of knowing the patient over a number of years, from previous visits to the medical department. He then will be able to detect any change in his speech, in his thinking, and in his conversation. Does the patient seem to have blocking in his thinking? Does he start to tell you something and then stop? Is his speech mixed up, or does he seem to range from topic to topic with no apparent connection? Is anger "in his speech"? Does he express fears? Does the patient seem to think that people are turning against him, that his supervisor or someone else seems to have it in for him? These are clues that he may have suspicious or paranoid tendencies. Does he think that people are talking about him? Usually in his conversation the patient will at some point mention these feelings. The physician may notice that the employee may cock his head as if he were listening to something. Hallucinations may be occurring at that time. The patient may state that he hears strange voices which upset him or bother him. One patient of mine told me in all seriousness that his teen-age son also heard the same voices and that they were interfering with his school work. He may feel that people are listening to him or that his department is wired to receive and to record what he says. Does he feel compelled to do certain things in a certain way? Does his conversation seem logical, relevant and coherent? Is the speech thick or altered in any way? Are there many pauses? Sometimes pauses last many minutes and the physician may have to ask the question again or rephrase it. Is the patient's mood reflected in his thinking? In the way he speaks? Is there much variation in emotional tone? In inflection in his speech?

The following are some thought processes with possible interpretations:

Thoughts	*Interpretations*
1. Confusion in thinking	1. Depressions, manic state, toxic or metabolic states, (hypoglycemic confusion) presenile and senile degenerative reactions, generalized arteriosclerosis, schizophrenic reaction, general paresis, taboparesis, brain tumor, brain abscess, subdural hematoma
2. Delusions (false beliefs)	2. Schizophrenia, paranoid states, depression, manic state, toxic and metabolic states, presenile and senile degeneration, generalized arteriosclerosis, general paresis, taboparesis, brain tumor, subdural hematoma, brain abscess
3. Hallucinations	3. Schizophrenia, paranoid reaction, depression, manic reaction, toxic and metabolic reaction, presenile and senile degeneration, generalized arteriosclerosis, general paresis, taboparesis, brain tumor, brain abscess

Thoughts	*Interpretations*
4. Paranoid ideas	4. Paranoid reaction, schizophrenia, depressive reaction, manic reaction, toxic and metabolic reaction, presenile and senile degeneration, general paresis, taboparesis, brain tumor, brain abscess
5. Obsessions, compulsions	5. Obsessive-compulsive reaction.
6. Depressive and suicidal thoughts	6. Depressive reaction, brain tumor, brain abscess, toxic and metabolic reactions, schizophrenic reaction, general paresis, taboparesis
7. Anxious thoughts, worry, concern	7. Anxiety reaction, long-standing neurotic reaction to life
8. Fears of things, situations and people	8. Phobic reaction
9. Thoughts of inferiority, of inadequacy	9. Inadequate personality—lifelong
10. Perfectionistic thoughts and activity	10. Obsessive-compulsive personality —lifelong
11. Fears of killing loved ones	11. Neurotic reaction (anxiety, phobic reaction)
12. Fears of doing wrongful acts, of thinking wrongful thoughts, of forgetting to do the right acts (scrupulosity)	12. Obsessive-compulsive personality
13. Thoughts of unreality (thinks the world not real)	13. Schizoid personality, schizophrenia

Stream of Thought

Here, I shall discuss only the form of how the patient talks, i.e., how he says it.

Form	*Interpretation*
1. Volubility (pressure of speech with logic and reason)	1. Manic and hypomanic reactions
2. Circumstantiality (goal is reached with much detail)	2. Rigid and compulsive personality
3. Flight of ideas (continuous stream of speech with chance associations causing many digressions from the topic being discussed)	3. Manic-depressive psychosis, manic type, hypomanic reaction

Form	Interpretations

4. Slowing of speech and mutism

4. Depression, severe (psychotic) depression, situational or reactive (neurotic) senile and presenile dementia, brain tumor (aphasia)
Mutism occurs in:
 1. Severe depression
 2. Complete indifference to environment
 3. Negativism
 4. Result of an hallucinatory command
 5. Complex-determined belief
 6. Difficulty in thinking

5. Blocking (sudden stoppage of speech, unexplained by patient, with resumption shortly)

5. Schizophrenic reaction, brain tumor (aphasia)

6. Deprivation of thought (severe blocking for a long time with apparently no mental content at all)

6. Schizophrenic reaction, severe depression, senile and presenile dementia, brain tumor, retarded mental states

7. Relevance (response of patient to questions are relevant, to the point, connected)

7. Usually occurs in depressions and schizophrenic reactions, anxiety reactions. *Irrelevance:* might occur in hypomanic and manic reactions, brain tumor, senile and presenile dementia, toxic reactions and metabolic reactions

8. Incoherence (disconnection between question asked and topic being discussed and response. Scattering and dilapidation of thinking and "word salad" represent severe types of incoherence)

8. Manic and hypomanic reactions, senile and presenile dementia, toxic and metabolic reactions such as spontaneous hypoglycemia with confusion

9. Perseveration (constant repetition of words or phrases)

9. Aphasic disorders in brain tumors, speech disorders as stuttering and stammering, schizophrenic reactions

Emotional Reaction (Affect)

Affect and mood are both used to denote the emotional state of the patient. Henderson states "Affect is the term of preference, as it has none of the popular connotations of "mood." Affect is difficult to define. The language of emotion is, in any case, very inadequate. Affect can, perhaps, be called the subject's inner feeling at a given moment, but this is not a definition."

The occupational physician will have observed the superficial expressions of the patient's affect or emotional reaction as he has taken a history and performed a physical examination. He will have noticed the facial expressions, the gestures, the general attitude and behavior of the patient. In examining more closely the emotions of the patient, the physician should try to analyze the situations producing the emotional reaction and attitude, whether it is due to on-the-job or off-the-job causes. We should always be thoughtful of the patient's feelings when we ask about his emotions. To an obviously depressed patient, we should not ask "Are you happy?" It would be more considerate to ask general questions such as "Tell me, how do you feel today?" or "How have your spirits been lately?" and follow this up with "Why do you suppose you have felt this way?" and "What have you been worrying about?" The patient may be asked to tell his story in his own way, while the physician should try to keep the patient to the topic with a minimum of questioning until his story has been detailed completely. In this way, the patient begins to realize that the physician is really interested in him and a genuine positive relationship develops which can mean much in the future course of the patient's troubles. Our questions should, of course, be dictated by common sense and should be used only to keep the patient to the topic at hand, without suggesting things. We are interested in what the patient has to say spontaneously because his verbalization represents what is on his mind and what has been troubling him. We do not wish to disturb him in his train of thought.

In questioning the patient about his emotional feelings, we should keep the following in mind, viz.:

1. Intensity of affect.
2. Does affect vary?
3. What seems to vary it during the examination?
4. Is affect in harmony with the ideas expressed?
5. What is the response to reassurance?
6. What is the predominant affect present during the examination? (such as elation, depression, suspicion, anger, fear, hate, anxiety, disharmony, panic, emotional indifference or apathy).

7. The affective state can be estimated even when the patient is unresponsive, by observing pallor, flushing, respiration, perspiration and the pulse and general gestures.

The following chart attempts to correlate certain neurologic and psychiatric conditions with various affective states as observed during the examination:

Emotional Reaction (Affect)	*Interpretations*
1. Depression	1. Depressive reaction (neurotic, reactive or situational) psychotic depressive reaction with mental and psychomotor retardation, brain tumor, brain abscess, toxic and metabolic reactions, presenile and senile degenerations, generalized arteriosclerosis, paresis, taboparesis, schizophrenia
2. Elation, (overly cheerful, joy, euphoria)	2. Manic reactions, irritability reactions, paresis, taboparesis, brain tumor, brain abscess, multiple sclerosis, toxic and metabolic reactions
3. Apathy, indifference	3. Schizophrenia reactions, severe depressions, melancholia
4. Belligerence, angriness, hostility	4. Psychopathic and paranoid personality reactions
5. Emotional deterioration (failure to show usual emotional responses)	5. Schizophrenia, presenile and senile dementia
6. Anxiety (fear of danger from within, anticipated physical illness, with symptoms and signs of fear)	6. Anxiety reactions, acute or chronic accompanying middleaged depressions, emotional instability, brain tumor
7. Apprehension (fear of external danger)	7. Anxiety reactions, paranoid reactions
8. Emotional instability or lability (fluctuations of affect without external cause)	8. Emotional instability (a type of pathologic personality)

General Knowledge

In the course of the conversation, the physician can usually size up the general knowledge of the patient. One must always keep in mind the nationality of the patient, the school level attained and the general experiences of the patient. The physician might ask general geographic and historical and mathematical questions to gain a broader insight into the general knowledge level of the patient. This data would aid in assessing the present mental status of the patient. If the patient is a college or high school graduate and at the present time cannot answer relatively simple questions about geography, history and mathematics, one should suspect that there has been some deterioration.

1. When was the Revolutionary War? Who was the American general in command?

2. Who fought the Civil War? Who was President of the Union at that time? Who was President of the Confederacy at that time?

3. How many states are there?

4. Where is London, Berlin, Rome, Washington, Chicago, Moscow, New Orleans, San Francisco, Minneapolis?

5. Who is President now? In World War I? in World War II?

6. Who is Governor of this state?

7. What is the capitol of France? Italy? New York? Massachusetts? California? Georgia? Texas?

8. Name the chief rivers of the United States.

9. What is the largest lake in the world? the highest mountain?

10. How much is 8 times 6? 4 times 18? Divide 24 by 6. Subtract 7 from 100 and keep on subtracting out loud.

Memory and Orientation

In getting a history of the complaints and the present illness, the physician will have a fine opportunity to test the recent and remote memory of the patient. As the patient relates his life in a chronological fashion, one can ascertain pretty well his ability to remember remote events. He should tell where and when he was born, when and where he left school and reasons why he left school. What further training did he have, when did he start his first job and where? What has been the longest time on one job? These questions will test remote memory fairly well. To *test recent memory* ask the following questions, viz.: What day is today? What did you have to eat for breakfast? For lunch? What did you do last night after work? What kind of work were you doing this morning before coming to see me? How did you get to work this morning? If the patient has forgotten what he had for breakfast, or what his wife's first name is, one should seek the cause of this memory difficulty. One may forget his breakfast because of a brain tumor, or because of cerebral degeneration. One may forget his wife's name because he has a strong emotional block to anything associated with his wife with whom he is having trouble at the present time. Of course he might have had some shock treatments recently which may be affecting his memory.

Memory	Interpretation
1. Poor recent memory	1. Senile and presenile dementia, a naturally poor rememberer, recent shock treatments, toxic and metabolic reactions, brain tumor, brain abscess, acute schizophrenic reaction.
2. Poor remote memory	2. A naturally poor rememberer. acute depression, acute schizophrenic reaction

To *test power of retention*, ask the patient to remember certain data which the examiner gives to him, such as: a street number, name of a person, name of a vegetable or fruit, or an object. A few minutes later, or an hour later, one may ask the patient to recall these data. Giving the patient word pairs also tests the power of retention, such as: nose — face; cigar — tobacco; ocean — brook; shrimp — whale; cabbage — squash; etc. The patient is asked to repeat these word pairs to familiarize himself with them and then the examiner gives the stimulus word to the patient.

Memory	Interpretation
3. Poor power of retention	3. Senile and presenile dementia, poor native intelligence, confusion due to toxic and metabolic reactions, acute depression, acute schizophrenic reactions

To *test orientation* one should ask the patient if he knows who he is, where he is, what time of day it is, what day of the week, what day of the month, of the year, etc.

Memory	Interpretation
4. Disordered interpretations as to time, person, and place	4. Confusional state, deep depression, acute and chronic schizophrenic processes, organic disease of the brain such as presenile and senile dementia, brain tumor, shock therapy, etc.

General Intelligence

This can usually be estimated by the general responses of the patient, as the conversation proceeds. One might ask the difference between idleness and laziness, a lie and a mistake, character and reputation. These responses would give a general idea of the intellectual level. Further tests for intelligence could be carried on later if necessary by those persons to whom the patient would be referred. One might use the Kent Emergency 10 Minute Test to estimate roughly the intelligence or age level of the patient (see end of chapter).[1]

Insight and Judgement

The occupational physician should try to assess how much the patient realizes his own condition. Questions such as the following might be asked, viz:

1. Do you think that you are ill?
2. Do you think that you are emotionally upset?
3. What do you think caused your trouble?
4. Do you think that things outside of you have caused your trouble?
5. Do you think that your ideas could be caused by a disturbed imagination?
6. What do you think might be done for you?
7. What is your judgement about this whole situation?

Many times people who are emotionally upset and who have physical symptoms will not admit the emotional origin of their troubles. The paranoid persons will project these things onto the environment. The inadequate person with immaturity traits will not have any idea but simply say that these are the bodily symptoms from which I suffer. One should know how these people look upon their illness as a guide to therapy. The depressed person thinks that all is lost and his judgement and insight are severely crippled by the depressed emotional state. The elated, happy, manic person does not think that anything is wrong — he is not sick.

Mental Mechanisms

The occupational physician would do well to be familiar with some of the thinking and a few of the mental mechanisms or processes which seem to be operating in all of us from time to time. This knowledge might enable him to understand his patient more thoroughly. I shall attempt only a brief description of these at this time. A fuller description can be found in textbooks of psychiatry. What I have written below is generally accepted, but naturally there are some people who will disagree with any definition.

1. "Abnormal" mental mechanisms differ in degree only from the normal. All of us have the same basic mechanisms.

2. Every "normal" or "average" person is neurotic at times, and every neurotic has much that is normal in him.

3. Much of the behavior and thinking is due to inner mental processes of which the patient is unaware.

4. Each mental process is determined by a preceding mental process, according to the *law of psychic determinism*. Every thought, action, feeling or gesture has a reason. Everything is determined.

5. Each mistake in speaking, in behaving, in remembering, is important and has a reason which may be buried by repression, conflicts, etc. Nothing is left to chance.

6. *Unconscious* processes play a large part in our mental life—conscious processes play only a small part.

7. The *unconscious* consists of previous impressions and memories and is a vital, dynamic, living system of mental processes.

8. *Conscious mental processes* obey laws of logic, relate to reality and time. *Unconscious mental processes* do not obey laws of logic, do not relate to time and reality.

9. *The pleasure-pain principle* guides the unconscious. The pleasure-pain principle guides many of our thoughts, actions and feelings, if we would be honest with ourselves.

10. The *unconscious* strives to express itself constantly, as it is charged with the energy derived from the instincts.

11. *Unconscious processes* influence behavior.

12. A *complex* is a group of ideas charged with emotion. The ideas have been deposited in the unconscious since childhood.

Title	*Definition*	*Functions*
13. Complex	13. A group of ideas charged with emotion — buried deeply in the unconscious. These ideas cannot reach consciousness as they conflict with principles of reality, conduct and belief	13. Affects behavior directly if it becomes conscious and indirectly if it cannot

14. Repression	14. An unconscious mechanism by which complexes (unconscious ideas) are prevented from reaching consciousness	14. Prevents unconscious ideas from reaching consciousness and prevents inner conflicts from incongruous ideas and actions
15. Consciousness	15. A "Sense organ" according to Freud	15. Recevies impressions from the outer world of reality and from the complexes (emotionally toned ideas) of the unconscious
16. The censor	16. Determines which emotionally toned ideas (complexes) will be admitted to the preconscious or conscious, or repressed to the unconscious	16. The censor determines if the complexes are compatible with reality. This is based on whether or not their admission will give pleasure or pain to the person
17. Displacement of affect	17. If a complex cannot reach consciousness, its emotion may be attached to another complex which can pass the censor, giving rise often to unexplainable conduct	17. A method to disguise painful or unpleasant affects
18. Projection	18. Occurs when the repressed complex is regarded as belonging to someone else. A person who has stolen thinks others are thieves	18. To protect the person against his own painful complexes
19. Dissociation	19. The ability of complexes to reside side by side in the unconscious without conflict. Thus ideas completely opposed to each other may be expressed, such as love and hate, peace and war, and the patient will not see any contradiction	19. To avoid conflict between the complexes

Title	Definition	Functions
20. Ego	20. Develops early in life as the first differentiation of the mind. It changes often during life as it balances the demands of instincts, conscience and the outer world	20. (1) The testing of reality (2) The recognition of the world outside and of the laws by which this world is governed (3) The modification of the demands of instinct which are unreasonable, insistent and immediate, so as to fit the demands of reality
21. Superego	21. Derived from ego and instincts. It comprises an ideal picture of oneself— a self-critical capacity, and conscience proper. These three faculties are the source of guilt	21. Acts as the conscience and critic of the individual
22. Denial	22. The unconscious denial of an observation	22. To avoid anxiety and pain
23. Regression	23. A slipping back into earlier habits and methods of doing things	23. To become dependent again on those around one
24. Sublimation	24. Is the process by which sexual energy is converted into constructive activity	24. To use sexual energy for other than sexual purposes
25. Conversion	25. Is an abnormal hysterical symptom which serves a defense purpose	25. To convert mental energy into a bodily symptom
26. Obsession	26. Is a recurrent thought that appears out of context, so that it baffles the patient and the casual observer	26. A defense against some aggressive thoughts
27. Transference	27. Directing or transfering to the physician of the patient's feelings and thoughts that have their origin in his relations with other persons, particularly those who are or have been close to him	27. Transference becomes the central theme in analysis, as the patient's feelings toward the physician call up the patient's past

The following is the Kent Oral Test which was referred to in the section on General Intelligence.[1]

Addenda II

Kent Ten Minute Oral Test

1. What are houses made of? One point for each item up to four   4
2. What is money made of?   Paper, four metals, one point each   5
3. Why does cork float on water? One point for light, lighter, or   3
   not so heavy. Two points for lighter than water which it displaces. Three points for lower specific gravity.
4. If the flag floats to the south, from what direction is the wind?   3
   Three points for north, no partial credits.
5. What is sand used for? One point for play or scrubbing. Two   4
   points for any construction use. Four points for glass. No cumulative.

Group II

6. Where do fishes live? Water or any body of water, one point.   1
7. What is candy made of? Two points for sugar, no additional   2
   credit for other items. One point each for two minor items.
8. What is the color of grass? Green, one point. Two points when   2
   brown or yellow is mentioned in addition to green.
9. How many days in a week? Two points when the answer is   2
   given easily, without hesitation. One point for counting correctly.
10. What does ice become when it melts? Water, one point.   1

Group III

11. How many minutes in an hour? Sixty, one point.   1
12. How many days in a month? 30 and 31, one point for each.   3
   One additional point for 28 or 29 referring specifically to February, no credit for 28 when it refers to four weeks.
13. Why is it colder at night than in the daytime? Two points for   3
   Sun goes down or other reference to lack of sun. Three points for rotation of earth. If child cannot answer at all, reverse the question: What makes it warmer in the daytime than at night? One point for correct answer to reversed question.
14. Tell me the name of some birds. One point each, up to four.   4
   If child stops with one, encourage him to go on.
15. Now the name of some fishes. One point each up to four.   4

Group IV

16. At what time of day is your shadow shortest? Noon, three points.   3
17. Give me the names of some large cities? One point each, up   4
   to four. If any state be mentioned as a city, New York is to be counted as a state unless given specifically as New York City.

18. What is paper made of? Wood, rags, cornstalks, one point each.　3
19. How many stripes in the flag? Thirteen, two points. A subject　2
who respond 48 should have his attention called to the mistake
and be permitted to try again. If he responds 7 it should be
made clear that both red and white stripes are included.
20. Whose picture is on a two cent stamp? Washington, two points.　2
Additional point for additional mention of special issue, but no
credit unless Washington is named.

Group V

21. What is the difference between a cable and a chain? Four　4
points for clear distinction between continuous strands and de-
tached links. One point for "chain has links." Two or three
points for intermediate distinction in use or material.
22. The stars are larger than the moon. Why does the moon look　4
larger? One point for 'Moon is lower down.' Three points for
closer or near to the earth. Four points for a generalized statement that a nearer object looks larger than a more distant one.
23. What metal is attracted by a magnet? Four for iron, two for　4
steel.
24. What is electricity used for? One point for light, heat, power.　4
One additional point for any other use, such as x-ray, telephone,
telegraph, radio. No cumulative for three used.
25. If your shadow points to the northeast, where is the sun? South-　4
west, four point. No partial credits.

Age	Points	Age	Points	Age	Points
Group 1, 2, 3		Group 1, 3, 4		Group 1, 4, 5	
6	2-7	8	15-20	9	19-22
7	8-13	9	21-25	10	23-26
8	14-20	10	26-29	11	27-30
9	21-26	11	30-33	12	31-34
10	27-31	12	34-36	13	35-38
11	32 up	13	37-39	14	39-42
		14	40-43	14 plus	43 up
		14 plus	44 up		

REFERENCE

1. Kent, G. H.: Oral Test for Emergency Use in Clinics. Mental Measurement Monographs. No. 9: Baltimore, Williams & Wilkins, 1932.

14. *Psychiatric Diagnostic Reminders*

FOLLOWING HIS PSYCHIATRIC EXAMINATION, the occupational physician should think of a diagnosis. For his purposes, a diagnosis will help him to decide on disposition, prognosis, therapy, and what information he will be able to relate to supervision so that the supervisor will be able to plan for the absence of the employee in the scheduling of work for his department. In the occupational setting, when one person is absent from work the plans and work schedule are altered, and the supervisor wants the Medical Department to tell him when he can expect to have his sick employee back again. The occupational physician wants to be able to decide whether he will be capable of treating the psychiatric condition of the employee or whether he should refer the patient to the psychiatrist in the company or the community. At times the employee states that he has no family doctor. In this case, the occupational physician must decide about referring the patient to the psychiatrist in the community if he feels that the condition is such that he is not qualified to care for the patient. The occupational physician of today is usually capable of treating the ordinary emotional upsets of the employee and also a few of the major psychiatric conditions. The occupational physician of the future will have had a broader training in the field of psychiatry than in the past or even in the present. He will be better able to diagnose a psychiatric condition as his training improves.

Detailed differential diagnostic points about the various psychiatric categories are probably not in order for the average occupational physician. It seems to me that the occupational physician might be able to decide whether one of the three following broad categories are present: (1) psychosis, (2) neurosis, (3) character or personality disorder. This would give him three broad categories for record purposes and also for his own thinking. If he is interested in further delineating the illness, he may do so under one of these three broad notologic entities. I realize that at times the occupational physician will simply satisfy himself that there is a psychiatric condition present and refer the patient to the community psychiatrist or the community clinic.

Actually, what the occupational physician wants to know in regard to making a diagnosis is the following:

1. What is the diagnosis, so that he will be able to do one of the following things: (a) treat the employee himself; (b) refer the patient to the family physician so that he may refer the patient to a psychiatrist of his choice; (c) refer the patient to a community psychiatrist or clinic if there is no family physician; (d) refer the patient to the family physician and discuss the psychiatric possibilities with the famly physician.

2. Estimate prognosis from the diagnosis.

To give the occupational physician a few pegs upon which he may hang a few diagnostic hats, I present the following diagnostic classifications (*modified for this purpose*) from the Manual of the International Statistical Classification of Disease, Injuries and Causes of Death, Sixth-Revision of the International Lists of Diseases and Causes of Death, World Health Organization, Geneva, Switzerland, 1949. Code numbers are omitted for simplicity's sake.

Psychoneurotic Disorders

1. Anxiety reaction without mention of somatic symptoms.
2. Hysterical reaction without mention of anxiety reaction.
3. Phobic reaction.
4. Obsessive-compulsive reaction.
5. Neurotic-depressive reaction.
6. Psychoneurosis with somatic symptoms affecting the circulatory system.
7. Psychoneurosis with somatic symptoms affecting the digestive system.
8. Psychoneurosis with somatic symptoms affecting others symptoms.
9. Psychoneurotic disorders, other, mixed, and unspecified types such as, hypochondriacal reaction, depersonalization, occupational neurosis, asthenic reaction, etc.

Disorders of Character, Behavior and Intelligence

1. Pathologic personality.
   schizoid, paranoid, cyclothymic, inadequate, antisocial, and asocial personality
   sexual deviation
2. Immature personality.
   emotional instability
   passive dependence
   aggresiveness

enuresis characterizing immature personality
other
3. Alcoholism.
4. Other drug addiction.
5. Primary childhood behavior disorders.
6. Mental deficiency.
7. Other and unspecified character, behavior and intelligence disorders.

Psychoses

1. Schizophrenic disorders (dementia praecox).
2. Manic-depressive reaction.
3. Involutional melancholia.
4. Paranoia and paranoid states.
5. Senile psychosis.
6. Presenile psychosis.
7. Psychosis with cerebral arteriosclerosis.
8. Alcoholic psychosis.
9. Psychosis of other demonstrable etiology, resulting from brain tumor, epilepsy, etc.
10. Other and unspecified psychoses.

Broadly speaking, the following are the main distinguishing characteristics of the above three principle psychiatric categories, viz.:

Psychoneurotic Disorders

1. Fairly good insight though symptoms are unconsciously determined.
2. He is maladjusted, though not antisocial.
3. His inner conflicts are in a struggle with the outer environment.
4. The ego is still strong enough to keep the personality intact and the unconscious inherent cravings repressed.
5. He is wrapped up with himself and his manifold psychological and physical symptoms — he is at war with himself and he wants the attention and sympathy of others.
6. Most neurotics are able to continue at work in spite of their symptoms, even though at a reduced performance level. Actually, they are better off working, as it seems that work becomes a form of therapy for them, although they will at times bitterly oppose the idea of working.
7. He knows he is ill but is sure it is due to a physical disorder.

Disorders of Character, Behavior and Intelligence

A. *Disorders of Character and Behavior*

1. Formerly known as psychopathic personality or psychopathic states.
2. May be predominantly aggressive, inadequate or creative.

3. Intelligent, selfish, very little consideration of others, never profits from punishment or experience, disrupts any group he may be in, is odd, conceited, irritating and exasperating.

4. May produce at work very well for a limited time but then fails.

5. Promises much and delivers little.

6. Loyal only to himself.

7. Becomes involved early and often with alcohol, drug and sexual patterns of behavior.

8. Becomes involved with the law from time to time.

B. *Disorders of Intelligence*

1. Evidences of defective intelligence from behavioral experiences on the job and from the results of intelligence tests.

Psychotic Disorders

1. Complete or partial loss of insight.

2. Has failed to adjust and has severed relations with society.

3. Has become antisocial or asocial.

4. The delusions and hallucinations are real to him.

5. Projection of his ideas onto the outer world.

6. Impairment of reason, judgement, logic and moral senses.

7. His unconscious is bared and has overcome the ego as the ego has not been able to repress any longer the powerful unconscious inherent strivings.

8. He does not think he is ill, the world is ill.

9. Most psychotics cannot work, though a few can work.

Malingering

Malingering must be mentioned for completeness sake, although it is not very common. The differential diagnosis between a neurosis and malingering is usually not very difficult. The following salient points about malingering should be remembered:

1. The aim is to deceive, for purposes of gain or to escape reality, etc.

2. Simulation of symptoms or disease which he has had or which he has observed others to have had.

3. Conscious production of symptoms as against unconscious production of symptoms in the neurotic.

4. The malingerer "overacts" or "overdoes it" and he is hard pressed to reproduce the same symptoms and signs over and over again over a long period of time. Observation of the suspected malingerer is then necessary over a prolonged period of time to catch him off guard.

5. He resents frequent complete examinations, whereas the neurotic and especially the hysteric welcomes them.

6. Several tests have been devised to detect malingering.

7. Symptoms do not resemble any type of neurosis or psychosis and change daily.

8. Signs of ill health absent.

9. Refusal of food is rare.

10. Onset of malingering is sudden.

11. Symptoms not maintained when he thinks he is unobserved.

CHARACTERISTICS OF PSYCHONEUROTIC DISORDERS

In the hope that the occupational physician might benefit from a capsule distillation of the main points of the various psychoneurotic disorders to aid him in putting his diagnostic mind in order, I venture the following, knowing full well that this procedure is always imperfect, at best. The differentiation of the neuroses one from another depends on one's point of view, and I suppose on what classification one is partial to using. However, practicality for the practicing occupational physician is my goal. Therefore, I shall outline briefly a few of the outstanding symptoms of each group. Pure psychoneurotic categories are not very common. Mixed psychoneurotic categories are common, and they show symptoms of the various groups, such as anxiety, phobias, depressive symptoms and hysterical manifestations (motor and sensory). In spite of this, I wish to mention the characteristics of the prototype, following the World Health Organization Classification outlined above.

Psychoneurotic Disorders

1. *Anxiety reaction,* without mention of somatic symptoms.

   a. Vague anxiety without any known cause.

   b. Palpitation.

   c. Fears of illness, death, cancer, impending disaster, etc.

   d. Restless, irritable, poor sleep and eating habits.

   e. Intellectual functioning undisturbed.

2. *Hysterical reaction,* without mention of anxiety reaction.

   a. Paroxysmal episodes of dramatic behavior, such as temper tantrums, screaming, "fainting," "throwing of fits" and various emotional outbursts.

   b. There may be disturbances of motor power, of sensation, of vision, of hearing, of speaking, of walking, etc., all of which do not conform to any organic neurologic pattern.

   c. Emotional instability and immaturity have been present in many cases.

d. Rarely occurs for the first time after forty years of age.

e. Symptoms represent an attempt to solve life's problems by escape from reality by aggressive or by passive means (paralyses, etc.)

3. *Phobic reaction*

a. A specific fear which the patient knows is silly but which he can do nothing about.

b. Main classes are: phobia of environment and phobia of disease.

c. Causes are usually deep in the unconscious.

d. An attempt to sidestep certain unpleasant situations in life.

e. Intellectual functioning undisturbed.

f. Behavior may be dictated by the respective phobia.

4. *Obsessive-compulsion reaction*

a. The patient is compelled to perform certain acts or to think certain thoughts or to say certain things.

b. Patient may feel that these compulsory acts are ridiculous, but he is powerless to do anything about them. The acts may occur alone or accompany the obsessive ideas.

c. The acts and ideas are defensive mechanisms against tabooed wishes and represent a compromise satisfaction of infantile wishes.

d. The affect from the repressed wish has been displaced to an idea which is acceptable to the consciousness of the individual.

e. These repressed wishes often have a sexual origin.

f. Patients often are most disturbed by these repetitive ideas and compulsive acts, developing sleeplessness, anxiety, fatigue, depression and multiple somatic complaints. At times, their daily behavior is paralyzed.

5. *Neurotic depressive reaction* (situational depressive reaction)

a. Caused by a situation in life.

b. Depression does not show retardation of thinking, of speech or of behavior and thus differs from psychotic depressive reaction.

c. Many somatic complaints accompany the feeling of depression.

d. Work may suffer as thinking, concentration and persistence of effort decline.

e. First symptoms may be physical.

6. *Psychoneuroses affecting various systems*

a. One or more systems may be involved in the neurotic reaction.

b. Symptoms usually secondary to the patient's reactions to his own ideas, attitudes and to life's situations.

c. Usually there have been previous episodes of neurotic reaction of one type or another.

d. Often a relative or friend has had similar disturbances of the same sort that the patient complains of — the patient identifies through his symptoms with the relative or friend.

CHARACTERISTICS OF THE VARIOUS TYPES OF DISORDERS

1. *Pathologic personality*

　a. Schizoid personality

　　1. History of aloofness, shyness, withdrawing from life.

　　2. More of a thinker than a doer — a dreamer.

　　3. Sensitive to people, to criticisms, and to life's blows.

　b. Paranoid personality.

　　1. Tendency constantly to suspect motives of people, to read between the lines, to look beyond the statements of people for hidden meanings, never to trust people implicitly, to doubt the intentions of people.

　　2. Never mixes well with people; remains aloof.

　　3. Is a poor group worker as he never can trust the people with whom he works.

　　4. Rigid personality — never relaxes.

　c. Cyclothymic personality

　　1. Mood swings from time to time — ups and downs.

　　2. Easily elated and easily depressed.

　　3. Usually good workers — effective producers on and off the job.

　　4. Elation and depression usually does not get out of hand — is not too profound — and so hospitalization is usually unnecessary. Time off from work occasionally is needed.

　d. Inadequate personality

　　1. Has never met situations adequately in life — many failures.

　　2. Depreciates self, often needs someone to lean on for decisions, for support, and for sustenance.

　　3. Constantly needs prodding to do things.

　　4. Is easily led by others — so may get into difficulty with the law and into social situations which may not be good.

　e. Antisocial

　　1. Is a law unto himself — conforms poorly or not at all to social customs, practices and laws.

　　2. Selfish, pleasure seeking, inconsiderate of others.

　　3. Profits not from punishment, from mistakes, or from advice.

　　4. In trouble with the law for many antisocial acts.

　　5. A poor worker, as he cannot conform, cannot work with others and rebels against authority (formerly known as constitutional psychopathic inferiority).

　f. Asocial personality

　　1. Prefers his own company to others — the lone wolf.

　　2. Usually does not have too many schizoid tendencies.

　　3. Makes a poor group worker but may make an excellent individual

worker if left alone and given resources and understanding.

4. May be a pathologic liar and show moral deficiency trends.

g. Sexual deviation

1. Includes exhibitionism, fetishism, homosexuality, pathologic sexuality, sadism and other forms of sexual deviation.

2. Many persons with these afflictions can work effectively and harmoniously as they have learned to control their tendencies. Some I know have been excellent workers.

2. *Immature personality*

a. Emotional instability

1. Marked lack of control over emotions, behavior.

2. Frequent episodes of impulsive and disruptive behavior.

3. Usually are poor workers though they can conform to the group and to regulations for a while — but, like children, they throw fits of temper when things don't go their way or they are criticized or suggestions made to them.

b. Passive dependency

1. Marked reliance on others for decisions, support and guidance.

2. May be a good group worker for a while if he can be handled wisely.

c. Aggressiveness

1. Excessive pushiness, of forcing his way and will on to others.

2. Very disruptive of life around him.

3. Selfish, greedy, inconsiderate, pleasure-seeking.

4. Usually cannot work well with groups — upsets departments and gets people disturbed — the social bacteria of the department.

d. Enuresis characterizing immature personality

1. Enuresis occurs as a symptom or as a solution to the problem of dealing with reality, on-the-job or off-the-job.

2. I have had patients with this condition who have been able to work satisfactorily. They are sensitive to any criticism of their work and have to be managed carefully.

3. *Alcoholism*

a. Acute — acute intoxication, alcoholic delirium, alcoholic hallucinosis, etc.

b. Chronic—long-standing problem with alcohol—poor insight, absenteeism and other job problems, family problems, and physical symptoms.

4. *Other Drug Addiction*

Usually occurs in individuals who are susceptible, weakwilled, dependent, passive and immature with feelings of inadequacy. They seem unable to face the realities and problems of life without leaning on a drug.

5. *Primary Childhood Behavior Disorders* — as tantrum, jealousy, masturbation and juvenile delinquency.

6. *Mental Deficiency*
   a. Various degrees, i.e., idiocy, imbecility, moron, borderline intelligence, mongolism.
7. *Other and Unspecified Character, Behavior and Intelligence Disorders*
   Specific learning defects, stammering and stuttering of nonorganic origin, other speech impediments of nonorganic origin. Acute situational adjustment.

CHARACTERISTICS OF PSYCHOTIC DISORDERS

1. *Schizophrenic disorders*
   a. Main subgroups for record purposes only—as occupational physicians will probably not be too interested in delineating these for all practical purposes on the job, viz.: Simple, hebephrenic, catatonic, paranoid, acute schizophrenic reaction, latent schizophrenia, schizoaffective psychosis.
   b. In the work place, whether it is the department store, the bank, the school, the voluntary agency or the factory, people with schizophrenic disorders can and do work. I have seen catatonics work well in between their acute catatonic episodes. Employees with acute schizo-affective crises and acute schizophrenic reaction will have to be hospitalized for their attack.
   c. Mainly, persons with a schizophrenic disorder of any type except the acute schizoaffective type show the following general characteristics: aloof, withdrawn, dreamer, shy, odd, sensitive, suspicious at times, cold, impulsive, poor emotional response.
2. *Manic-depressive reaction*
   a. Manic type
      1. Episodes of uncontrolled elation and behavior, poor judgement, insight and reasoning; patient has to be hospitalized to protect himself against his overactivity, and his irrational and illogical ideas.
      2. Previous history of episodes of overactivity.
   b. Circular type
      1. Alternating episodes of over- and underactivity, of elation and depression.
   c. Depressive type
      1. Episodes of profound depression with marked retardation of think-'ing, of action, delusions of the body systems, marked depreciatory feelings of self, suicidal ideas and attempts, poor sleep, poor appetite, and, at times, depressive stupor.
3. *Involutional melancholia*
   a. Depression with or without agitation occuring in the menopausal age period — in women in the fifth and sixth decades of life, and in men in the sixth and seventh decades, varies in degrees from mild to profound depres-

sion, depreciatory ideas, ideas of regret of the past, bemoans the future, delusions of the body, poor eating and sleeping habits, suicidal thoughts and attempts.

b. Mild cases may work and it may be therapeutic for them to do so.

4. *Paranoia and paranoid states*

a. Well systematized delusions of one or more ideas.

b. Otherwise, the actions and thoughts and feelings of these patients may seem quite average. It is only when the complex of ideas, around the paranoid trends are attached, is approached does the behavior of the patient become abnormal. Later in life, during aging, decompensations may occur and the patient loses control of the ideas and his behavior.

c. Most of these patients are able to work and to produce effectively. In fact, their colleagues may never know about these paranoid ideas unless they happen to be mentioned in a casual conversation. Stresses in life, fatigue and illness may cause a temporary decompensation.

5. *Senile psychoses*

a. Begin to occur in the seventh decade of life and later.

b. Memory difficulties, poor judgement, transitory confusional episodes, defective reasoning, depression, deviant sexual behavior, faulty personal hygiene, irritable, inconsiderate, a change of the personality for the worse, delusions and many bodily symptoms.

c. Work suffers because of the above symptoms, and sick leave is indicated.

6. *Presenile psychoses*

a. Similar symptoms and progress of the condition, but at an earlier age, usually in the fifth or sixth decade of life. Cerebral atrophy is found usually on pneumoencephalography.

7. *Psychosis with cerebral arteriosclerosis* (Organic brain disease)

a. Symptoms of cerebral arteriosclerosis occur along with the symptoms mentioned above in the presenile and senile psychoses. These may be due to minor and transitory strokes causing mild and transitory speech disturbances, weakness of an extremity, sensory changes in the face, arm or leg, visual defects, headaches, dizziness with hypertension.

b. These people can work for a time, but sooner or later it is necessary to put them on sick leave.

8. *Alcoholic psychosis*

a. Usually an alcoholic who develops a psychosis is not working at the time, as his heavy drinking precludes this. But the occupational physician is often called to the employee's home when such a development occurs.

b. The type of psychosis may vary, but it usually consists of hallucinations, delusions, confusion, disturbed behavior, with no appetite and poor nutrition, inability to sleep, etc. Hospitalization is necessary.

9. *Psychosis of other demonstrable etiology*
    a. This may occur in the course of a brain tumor, in an epileptic, in spontaneous hypoglycemia, acute infectious disease, poor nutritional states.
    b. Hospitalization is necessary.

PSYCHIATRIC DIAGNOSTIC REMINDERS

The author thought that a list of a few symptoms and signs with a discussion of what they might remind the physician of might be in order. This is not a textbook and the author recommends those who wish to read more of these psychiatric syndromes to consult the many good textbooks on psychiatry.

Symptom or Sign	*Interpretation*
1. Can't seem to get going in the morning.	1. Neurotic state — anxiety, depression or a mixed state.
2. I don't want to go to bed at midnight. I feel the best at night.	2. Neurotic state — anxiety, depression or a mixed state, or plain bad health habits.
3. I feel the women on the next bench are thinking of me when I see them laughing.	3. May be the development of paranoid trends.
4. When I see the women in the other end of the department talking, I think they're talking about me.	4. May be the development of paranoid trends.
5. When a patient recites a list of symptoms and states that they seem to have developed at a certain time.	5. Always ask what might have happened in the patient's life at the time the symptoms began. Usually there is some life's experience which triggered off the list of symptoms.
6. When physical conditions for the multiple complaints of patients have been ruled out, these symptoms have meaning.	6. In more than 85% of patients these symptoms have originated from off the job life's experiences, centering around the home and social life.
7. Headache, migraine, dizziness, vertigo, visual troubles, hearing difficulties, impairment of hearing in one or both ears.	7. One should always rule out neurologic diseases of the brain, such as brain tumor, subdural hematoma, brain abscess, if there has been a recent infection or some type of encephalitis.

Symptom or Sign

8. Difficulty in sleeping.

9. Ringing in the ears, noises in the head.

10. Worry over palpitation or pains in the chest when physical and laboratory tests and examinations have proved negative.

11. Worry about a particular organ or system of organs in the presence of no demonstrable physical condition.

12. Weakness, lassitude, apathy, tires easily on slightest effort.

13. Lump in the throat or difficulty in swallowing.

14. Episodes of diarrhea or constipation.

Interpretation

8. May be an early depressive reaction beginning, or it may be worry about on-the-job or off-the-job problems.

9. In young people, these symptoms often are those of an emotional upset, such as anxiety state, particularly. In older people, such as middle age and older, they may be the sign of arteriosclerotic processes in the inner ear. Otosclerosis also must be considered in young people who develop symptoms of tinnitus along with decrease in hearing.

10. Usually an anxiety state accompanied by many physical and emotional symptoms secondary to on-the-job or off-the-job problems.

11. An anxiety state based upon identification with some relative or friend who has had a similar disease in the past.

12. These may be the early signs of a depression if they have not occurred before. If the patient has had a lifelong history of asthenia and easy fatigueability and tiredness on slight effort, the possibility of a neurasthenic syndrome must be considered.

13. Usually conversion hysteria. There is something in the patient's life which he cannot swallow.

14. In the absence of any demonstrable pathology in the gastrointestinal system, usually due to emotional upsets such as anxiety or mild depression. When x-rays reveal a spastic colon, the cause must be sought for in the patient's life history and experience.

15. I have to be sure of everything at work and at home. I like to do things orderly and meticulously. Things must be in order.

15. An obsessive compulsive condition must be considered. A certain degree of this pattern of living is a virtue and worthwhile in any occupation, but it can become a vice and paralyze the functioning of the individual at work and at home.

16. I seem to think that the radio and the television are influencing my every action.

16. Probably the beginning of a paranoid pattern.

17. I have a dull pressure on the. top of my head, or I have a tight band around my head. and sometimes I have pressure in the back of my neck.

17. Usually a neurotic symptom indicative of an emotional upset over a life's experience.

18. Following a back injury, a patient develops a multiplicity of symptoms involving not only the chest, arms, neck and head.

18. Probably conversion hysterical symptoms developing in other parts of the body, possibly secondary to the back injury, but probably due to other factors in the life of the individual.

19. I see double in one eye.

19. Conversion hysteria.

20. My hand that I do all the work with goes numb from time to time and I get cramps in it and I can't do my work.

20. Usually a conversion hysteria which is commonly known as an occupational neurosis. This has meaning to the patient in relationship to the job or/and to some life's experiences outside of the job.

21. My eyelids twitch from time to time, or I have live flesh under my eyes.

21. Usually an anxiety state secondary to some problem on the job or off the job.

22. "I'm not an alcoholic," in an individual who is having alcoholic problems, and also the problem of absenteeism at work, and poor quality of work. "I can handle my drinking perfectly all right."

22. The individual is undoubtedly an alcoholic in the true sense of the word but has not been able to accept this idea.

23. I am very happy when Monday morning rolls around and I can go back to work. The boss lays my work out for me

23. In the field of occupational psychiatry, this syndrome is known as the *weekend neurosis*. These are people who cannot stand disorgani-

Symptom or Sign	*Interpretation*
and I know what I have to do during the day. Everything is on time: my coffee breaks, my lunch, etc.	zation in their lives and usually weekends at home are rather disorganized. These people love orderliness and have to have the day well planned ahead of time. There is a certain amount of obsessive compulsive tendencies in these persons.
24. Since my promotion, I have been all upset, depressed, nervous, can't eat or sleep, can't think right.	24. Promotion Depression. Patient has been promoted when he has not the ability for the new job or it is too early for his promotion — or he does *not wish* to be promoted. Management learns the hard way that some men do not wish to be promoted.

REFERENCES

1. Henderson, Sir David, and Gillespie, R. D.: Textbook of Psychiatry, ed. 7. London, Oxford University Press, 1950.
2. Sadler, W.: Modern Psychiatry. St. Louis, C. V. Mosby Company, 1945.

15.   *Psychiatric Treatment Reminders*

LONG-TERM PSYCHIATRIC TREATMENT, as psychiatrists understand it, will probably not be practiced by occupational physicians in any work setting. Psychiatrists on occupational medical staffs may practice a limited form of a generally accepted psychiatric therapy, viz., brief psychotherapy. *However, this monograph is written for the benefit of occupational physicians. Psychiatric treatment, therefore, will be limited in any occupational setting.* This does not preclude the occupational physician from utilizing certain psychiatric techniques which psychiatrists have devised.

An occupational physician who is interested in people and in helping them to understand themselves and their problems can do a creditable job in psychotherapy if he uses only a few of the techniques devised by psychiatrists. One important technique utilizes the *doctor-patient* relationship.

The doctor-patient relationship is basic to the understanding by the physician of the patient and his problem. It is also basic to the understanding by the patient of himself and his problem. In spite of the fact that insight therapy or uncovering therapy would not be suitable in any occupational setting, the occupational physician can help the patient to understand in a superficial sort of way what some of his immediate problems may be and what the patient might do to alleviate some of his problems. This psychotherapy has been termed brief psychotherapy and was used extensively in the military services during World War II. Occupational psychiatrists have been using this type of therapy in their various occupational medical practices.

The occupational physician, in order to practice this type of therapy, must understand himself, his prejudices, his impatience, his fears, his hostilities, as best he can. He also must learn to be somewhat passive during the interview. Sometimes it is asking too much of a physician to be a sympathetic, warm and understanding listener. Some physicians must be able to do something or else he feels he is not entering into the therapeutic relationship at all. The medical school in the nonpsychiatric courses teaches physicians to do something actively *to* patients; to order this, to apply this, change this, take this or that, perform exercises, take walks, soak the feet, apply hot applications, etc. But in psychotherapy the physician must sit and listen. Not only with his two ears, but also, as it has been sometimes mentioned, with the third ear. He must listen to what the patient is saying and also to what the patient is not saying. I suppose that one might call this the interview type of therapy, in which the physician sees the patient once, twice, three or four times and, because of his attitude of listening, the patient is able to spend time in ventilation. Time is of the essence in this kind of therapy. Here, I would like to quote some pertinent remarks on "Interviewing" by Bond, Flumerfelt and Bidder in the section on psychiatry in *The Specialties in General Practice* by Cecil and Conn.[1]

INTERVIEWING

The psychiatrist is often a little surprised to hear other physicians express amazement at the apparent ease with which he obtains information from his patients. There are a few simple things that psychiatrists automatically do not do in order to create an atmosphere that allows people to confide in them — for, as a matter of fact, some kind of positive interference on the physician's part is usually necessary to *prevent* the patients' confessions. The psychiatrist, like the priest, has learned the magic of the closed door in obtaining confidential information in an atmosphere of utmost privacy.

Contrast with the method of the psychiatrist the way in which many a physician's office is run, with perhaps both doors open, with an office nurse running in and out, and with many telephone interruptions, during which the doctor perhaps speaks in exasperation or with an unusual degree of solicitude, taking up time which the patient feels for the moment should belong to him. For the doctor to answer a phone call just when a patient is on the verge of making an intimate disclosure and then to turn to the patient with an 'AH-now-let's-see-where-were-we' remark, is as effective a way of throwing cold water on a sensitive person as one could hope to find.

Ward rounds furnish another example of an atmosphere which does not inspire confidence. The doctor is usually well protected by a bevy of nurses, a resident, an interne or two, and perhaps some medical students. He sweeps into the room with a 'how-are-we-today' question, often answers it himself, and is on his way.

But even in the closed room with complete privacy there are things which, if done, will effectively prevent a patient from talking. For the doctor to sit plainly evidencing his impatience; to counter every confession from the patient with one of his own —'Why, the same thing happened to me!'; to reassure the patient too quickly before it is clear whether he is reassuring him about the correct thing (and this is often a difficult matter to decide); to laugh off the patient's symptoms; to side violently either with or against the patient; to talk all the time himself; to look bored; to write down every word that the patient says; to feel the urgency of making a decision 'for the patient's sake' before one is clear in his own mind; to be intolerant of the patient's silences — all these stand in the way of easy communication on the part of the patient. (It is not always necessary, of course, for a doctor to obtain extremely personal information from the patient, but he should be able to do so if the situation warrants.)

To promote the securing of information from the patient, the doctor should endeavor to create an atmosphere that is free from pressure or impatience, free from criticism or condemnation. It should be an atmosphere of friendliness, with respect on both sides. Students, and many physicians too, find themselves acutely uncomfortable at first in such situations and consequently do too much of the talking themselves. They are beset with the question, 'What can I say to the patient?' rather than with the more appropriate reflection, 'I wonder what he'll tell me today.' Practice builds confidence in this matter. Usually at the beginning, i.e., for several visits, the doctor is puzzled as to diagnosis and treatment. Most patients respond favorably if the doctor states frankly that he is as yet unable to make a diagnosis, but continues to show an interest in them and asks them to come back to discuss their problems further. It is far better for the doctor to proceed in this manner than to become routine in prescription-giving or to be forced into premature decisions.

One of the most effective tools that psychiatrists, as well as a great many other physicians, use routinely is silence. It is actually amazing how few direct questions a doctor needs to ask, how little he needs to say himself to the majority of his patients. A particularly strategic time for silence on the physician's part is when the patient has been talking along and then suddenly falls silent. Usually this sudden silence means that the patient has just thought of something which he is reluctant to tell. The best way to obtain this important information is for the doctor to meet the patient's silence with an expectant silence of his own. At such times the patient will welcome a digression, and anything the doctor may say the patient will seize upon in an effort to avoid talking about what is actually pertinent to his problem. In most instances, the physician should not allow such digressions. Silence on the doctor's part is a tacit way of saying also that the problem belongs to the patient and that information about it must come from him. In other words, silence puts pressure upon the patient. This technical device, like every other, can of course be overdone.

RELATIONSHIP BETWEEN PHYSICIAN AND PATIENT

Bond et al. declare that a physician does not have to see too many patients before he realizes that the feelings which the patient has toward him are the bridge over which communications travel. "When the patient falls silent, his silence is always due to some consideration he may have in regard to the physician." Often, such thoughts as, "Do I trust the doctor enough to tell him this?" "Will he think too badly of me if I tell him that?" or it may be something like this, viz: "I should not have told him what I did last week," "Well, I'll never tell him that."

Further on in their book, Bond et al. state in essence more sound facts about this matter, viz.:

The patient's feelings toward the physician begin before he appears in the doctor's office. He usually is referred by an expatient, a friend of an expatient or by a physician, so he arrives for the first visit with a preconceived idea that the physician has superior ability. For the first few moments of the first visit the patient is sizing up the physician and comparing his preconceived idea of the physician with the facts as he sees the physician, watches the physician's behaviour, emotions, attitudes, etc. as the physician takes a history. Since illness is a regression, the patient will usually tend to develop a dependence on the physician and at times almost a reverence for the physician. The patient's feelings toward the physician are one of the strongest sources of help the physician has to draw on for through this relationship is established the confidence which makes management easy.

The physician should keep this advantage of a positive physician-patient relationship by behaving in a way that does not undermine this relationship or give the patient the feeling that the physician is incompetent.

A feeling of incompetence could be communicated to the patient by:

1. Appearing confused about the diagnosis.
2. Telling the patient he is not sure what the treatment should be.
3. Figuratively scratching and shaking his head over every historical item or physical finding.
4. Complaining to the patient in his presence of the difficulties that patient's illness causes him (the physician).
5. Not being sure of the results of the examinations he makes.
6. Communicating his own anxiety to the anxious patient in worried facial expressions and fruitlessly repeated tests.

7. **Being** overcautious in repeating tests for fear of missing obscure physical findings.

8. **Being** reticent to explore the patient's emotional life.

One example may reveal the special significance of the patient-physician relationship. This is taken from the writing of Bond et al.

An excellent but somewhat shy physician had been giving quinidine to a woman patient with paroxysmal atrial fibrillation. On one visit he noticed that she seemed quite upset and he felt well satisfied with himself because he was able to get her out of the office before she commenced crying. Later the woman's husband phoned to the doctor and scolded him for having in his waiting room a magazine article which vigorously attacked the use of quinidine as a drug and which stated that its dangers far outweighed its usefulness. This phone call saved the doctor his patient. The woman had felt tricked by someone in whom she had originally felt the greatest confidence.

In explaining this case Bond et al. state the following:

This incident illustrates the common error of reticence. If the physician upon noticing his patient's anxiety, had closed the door behind her and remarked calmly, "You seem somewhat upset today," undoubtedly the grateful patient would have told him what was on her mind and he could have reassured her. Usually it is a good idea to let the patient give a full account of his doubts and worries before the doctor attempts to reassure him.

Ocassionally, a patient will show much hostility to the physician in many ways. The physician should try to understand this hostility. What does it mean anyway? The physician should understand that the patient is not personalizing his hostility to him, that is to the physician himself. He is using the physician as a symbol which represents something in the patient's past life. Instead of kicking the patient out of the office with the admonition, "Don't darken my threshold again if you're going to behave like that," the physician should seize on this opportunity to find out what is back of this hostility. *There is always a meaning to behavior.*

The occupational physician who feels that he does not have time to spend with the patients in a few sessions should probably not attempt this type of therapy. An employee who makes repeated trips to the dispensary to see the nurse or the doctor for a few moments, to get some pills or other medicine for his symptoms, probably aggregates, over the course of a year, many more minutes in total than if the patient had spent 30 minutes or more with the doctor on one, two, three or four occasions. The oft-repeated statement of the employee to the physician who does take time to listen to the story is as follows: "Well, you know, doctor, this is the first time that any doctor has ever taken the time to listen to my story." The physician many times will state that he has not got the time to listen to these neurotics go on about their symptoms. These patients do have a story to tell, and there is always a meaning behind their story, their behavior, their feelings, their thinking, their inclinations, their gestures, etc.

For an effective doctor-patient relationship, the physician must himself assume a posture of accepting the patient for what he is, for what he does, for what he says, for what he feels, and for what he thinks. The physician must have an open mind about the whole situation. He must never make up his mind ahead of time. He must translate into the patient the idea that he, the physician, is ready to listen and that he is ready to help the patient to understand himself and his problem. This type of interview, of course, should only be undertaken when the physician has first taken a history, done a physical and a neurologic examination and has assured the patient that, as far as he is concerned, there is no physical condition present. Laboratory tests may have to be made in order to supplement the clinical findings on examination. It is then up to the physician to assure the patient that, as far as he can tell, there is nothing organically wrong.

The doctor may then state to the patient that many times emotional things, tensions, worry, emotional upsets and life's situations, will produce bodily symptoms. He may ask the patient to tell him more about himself. This may take the form of asking the patient to tell him when these symptoms began and what might have happened in his life when these symptoms began. Some patients talk readily and others do not. The physician may have to prod the patient from time to time by asking pertinent questions. When did the patient first notice these symptoms? Where did it seem to occur for the first time? In what setting was the patient in at the time the symptoms occurred, etc. He might also inquire about the family life of the patient. What does the family consist of? Have other members of the family ever had this condition before? Where did the patient go to school? In what was the patient interested in life? What are the patient's goals? Why is the patient working at this particular job? Did he have any ambitions to improve himself at work? What does the wife think about the patient's complaints? What is the wife's state of health? The purpose of the physician's asking pertinent questions such as the above is to open up new avenues of approach to the problem.

It is always surprising to the physician to find relevant material pouring forth from the patient when a certain area of the patient's life is exposed. At times, the physician least expects to find any relevant material from the opening up of a certain area. The physician must rely on the verbal productions of the patient, as well as the nonverbal manifestations, such as intonations of voice, gestures, emotional expressions of the face, movements of the body in the chair, the emotional reactions of the patient, signs of restlessness, irritability, anger, etc. Many times what the patient doesn't say, or what he almost says, is more important than what he does say. Once the patient realizes that the physician is ready to sit back and to listen and to help, he is usually ready to talk. This may not occur in the first or the second interview; but sooner or later the patient begins to realize that he can have confidence in the doctor, and that the doctor is ready and willing to help.

The physician must be able to accept whatever the patient says, even if the substance of the patient's remarks is directed against the doctor, or the patient's supervision, or the company as a whole. Expressions of anger, hostility, bitterness, resentment, etc., must be accepted as material to be studied and investigated. There is always meaning behind the patient's behavior, thoughts and feelings. The physician must never lose sight of this. Within his patient is the explanation of the patient's behavior. If the patient seems to warm up to the physician, likes him, patronizes him, or even praises him, we may label this a positive relationship.

There may be some reasons why this relationship has been established in a positive way. The physician is always being identified with somebody in the patient's life. If the physician reminds the patient of somebody that the patient has always admired and liked, then it will be a positive relationship. On the contrary, if the physician reminds the patient of somebody whom he does not like, then it may very well be a negative relationship. At any rate, there is meaning in these relationships. The doctor must be ready, willing and able to accept a negative relationship and not kick back at the patient, or kick the patient out of of the office because the patient has dared to criticize the doctor or the company or the supervision or somebody else.

The occupational physician must learn to control his emotions, his facial expressions, his behavior and his tongue. He should develop two big ears and one small mouth. The physician may disapprove heartily of many of the things that the patient says or has done or is thinking of doing or is feeling. The physician can lead the patient to discussing these various thoughts, feelings and actions so that the patient comes to a conclusion himself as to what he should or should not say or do or think. In this way, the patient makes his own decisions and is thereby strengthened by so doing. It is always a temptation for the physician to say, "I think you should do this or that," or "I wouldn't do this." This fosters further dependency of the patient upon the physician. We must realize that patients lean on the physician from time to time when troubles arrive. This is known as the dependency relationship, which occurs in all doctor-patient relationships. Especially in the field of the emotions, patients will become quite emotionally dependent upon the physician for long periods of time, until they are able to stand on their own two feet and manage their own emotional lives.

Often, it may help the patient to talk more freely and also to help the physician control his emotions easier if the physician sits with his back slightly towards the patient and look in a direction away from the patient. The physician must always explain this maneuver to the patient so he does not think the physician is not listening. The physician can make a simple statement that he thought that possibly the patient would be able to talk more freely if the doctor looked away from the patient. If tears develop during the interview, the patient should be allowed to cry it out. The doctor should make no comment about this, but deftly and silently he can place a supply of tissues on the desk within reach of the patient. Crying is a good form and an effective form of emotional expression, and often the patient feels much better after it is over. When pauses develop in the patient's recital of his problems, the doctor should respect these pauses. If the pause goes on for too many minutes, the doctor might simply ask the question, "What are you thinking about now?" This usually gets the patient off again, possibly on another topic. When the end of the first interview is at hand, the physician states simply and casually something about the fact that much ground has been covered today and that in the next interview, for which an appointment is made, they will take up where they left off. The doctor might even suggest that, in the interim, the patient might like to jot down some things he might have forgotten to bring out during the first interview. The physician can suggest that the patient bring in the list of things to the next interview and use them as a springboard for future discussions.

In a surprisingly large number of cases, the patient will return for the second interview with the remark that he feels much better and that just getting some of these things off his chest has helped. There will undoubtedly be new topics to discuss and also it may be necessary to go over the things that were brought up in the first interview. Over the course of a few interviews, the patient may begin to feel better and it may seem wise to cut off therapy at this juncture. The occupational physician always has to decide whether he should attempt this short form of therapy with his patient or not. Certainly the patient should be referred back to the patient's family physician in the community if this is possible. The family physician may wish to carry on this form of brief psychotherapy himself. He should certainly be allowed the opportunity to do so. When the patient states that he has no family physician and would like to have the occupational physician take care of his problems, then the occupational physician must decide whether he feels capable to go ahead. There will be situations in which there is no family physician available in the community, and here again, the occupational physician must decide whether he wants to carry on this type of therapy. As the physician has seen the patient in a few interviews, he then will have an opportunity to decide whether he feels himself capable of carrying on. If the patient does not seem to improve, or seems to get worse, if the symptoms seem to be rather well fixed, profound or disabling to the patient as far as his work or his living is concerned, the occupational physician must decide about referring the patient to a community psychiatrist. There will be some occupational physicians in some areas of the country who will always refer these patients to the psychiatrist in the community, to a psychiatric clinic in the community, or to a distant psychiatric facility. He may decide that he does not wish to handle this type of case.

As to various medicines to help the patient over the hump in his problem, the occupational physician has a wide range of choice among the antidepressants, tranquilizers, sedatives and hypnotics. There are some psychiatrists who state that, if the patient's problems seem to be mostly emotional, the physician should never give any medicine. I believe that the doctor should give suitable medicine to help the patient temporarily with his distressing symptoms. The physician can explain that the medicines by themselves cannot cure the patient from his symtoms, but will only help him to feel better so that he will be better able to grapple with his emotional problems. I think that this is a defensible practice and should be followed. There will be some patients who will latch on to the medicine as another crutch, and the physician must be aware of this and gradually withdraw the medicine as the patient improves.

Certainly, if the patient develops severe depressive symptoms with suicidal thoughts, develops severe eating problems and poor nutrition, cannot sleep, and seems to be literally falling apart, then certainly the occupational physician must take the cue and refer the patient to a psychiatrist. Hospitalization and further treatment may be necessary in these cases. The occupational physician who would like to interest himself further in psychiatric matters that might pertain to his occupational practice might read one or more of the suggested books listed at the end of this chapter.

The occupational physician should familiarize himself with committment procedures in the community in which he works. Occasions may develop within his work setting whereby an employee becomes acutely ill and disturbed and needs hospitalization immediately. The family physician or the psychiatrist might be able to handle this situation for the occupational physician. In those instances in which there is no family physician or he is unavailable, or there is no psychiatrist available in the community, the occupational physician may have to take steps to insure the immediate and proper handling of the patient. In some states, facilities are set up whereby an obviously mentally disturbed patient can be admitted without committment procedures to a hospital facility for a period of observation. At any rate, the occupational physician should know ahead of time just what the procedures are, what the facilities are, and whom to call in case of an emergency.

The occupational physician should also familiarize himself with the various psychiatric facilities and agencies and clinics in the community in which he works.

At the start of the interview in which the patient is encouraged to talk about his problems, the physician should point out to the patient that anything he says is confidential. The author keeps notes on 5 x 8 cards which are filed in a locked file in each of the various plants in which he works. This encourages the patient to talk at will, as they know that all of their remarks are kept confidential and none will be placed on a general medical record. During the interview the physician need not make a word by word report of what the patient says. If he does, he will be unable to listen to the patient properly. General notes to cover the patient's story should be placed on the card, sufficient to recall to the physician's mind later on what the entire story is.

If a job problem seems to be included in the patient's recital of his problem, the physician may wish to talk with somebody in the personnel department, industrial relations department or supervision, or some other person in the company. This should not be done, of course, unless the patient is asked by the physician if the patient would mind if the physician talked with so and so about his problem. If the patient refuses, then there the matter rests. The physician later on in future interviews might bring up the matter again. Only if the patient assents to the physician's talking to anybody should any talking be done. Transferring a patient from one department to another in an attempt to solve his problems should not be done unless there is a sound basis for the transfer. Manipulative environmental therapy should only be attempted when there is a sound basis. The team approach in the handling of a worker's problem which seems to stem from the job is a sound approach. This team may consist of the medical department, supervisory department, industrial relations department, and any other departments that may be affected by the problem of the patient. The physician should keep his counsel at all costs.

THE REFERRAL TO A PSYCHIATRIST

When an occupational physician can find no physical basis for the symptoms, he might say to the patient: "After listening to your troubles and examining you thoroughly, I can find no physical basis for your symptoms. It may be that emotional factors may be causing some of your symptoms. Maybe you might tell me something more about your life — your home, your job and yourself, etc." The point is that the patient should be allowed to talk about himself. After a few sessions, the physician may conclude that a psychiatrist should handle the case. He may then say to the patient, "You and I have talked about the possibility of emotions causing your symptoms. I think it would be better for you if a physician who has had special training in the emotions, might see you." In this way, the patient is referred to a psychiatrist without too much trauma. If the patient should ask if the doctor is a psychiatrist, one should answer, "Yes, he is a psychiatrist. He has studied about nerves and emotions."

REFERENCES

1. Cecil, R. L., and Conn, H. F.: The Specialties in General Practice, ed. 2. Philadelphia and London, W. B. Saunders Co., 1957.
2. Ross, T. A.: The Common Neuroses, ed. 2. Baltimore, Williams and Wilkins Co., 1937.
3. Henderson, Sir David, and Gillespie; The Late R. D.: Textbook of Psychiatry, ed. 7. New York, Oxford University Press, 1950.
4. Noyes, A. P.: Modern Clinical Psychiatry. Philadelphia, W. B. Saunders Co., 1953.
5. Ewalt, J. R., Strecker, E. A., Ebaugh, F. A.: Practical Clinical Psychiatry. New York, Blakiston, 1957.
6. Henderson, Sir David: Psychopathic States. London, Chapman and Hall, Ltd., 1939.
7. Witmer, Helen, Ed.: Teaching Psychotherapeutic Medicine. New York, The Commonwealth Fund, 1947.
8. Hart, B.: The Psychology of Insanity, ed. 4. New York, The MacMillan Company, 1944.
9. Crichton-Miller, H.: Psychoanalysis and Its Derivatives, ed. 2. New York, Oxford University Press, 1947.
10. Wechsler, I. S.: The Neuroses. Philadelphia, W. B. Saunders Co., 1929.

16. *Optimum Time Off for Psychiatric Disabilities*

THE FOLLOWING REMARKS, culled from an address by the author, may guide the occupational physician in determining when his patient with a psychiatric disability might return to work. I shall discuss only the following psychiatric conditions as they are the most common in an occupational setting, viz.:

1. Anxiety reactions
2. Neurotic-depressive reactions
3. Schizophrenic reactions
4. Manic-depressive reactions
5. Paranoid reactions
6. Involutional reactions

Anxiety Reaction

The anxiety states comprise the bulk of the psychiatric conditions in community and industrial medical practice. Although most of the people that psychiatrists see in industry are so-called "normal" people, they do have troubles and most of these troubles are on an anxiety basis. These are troubled workers. Most of their troubles come from off the job and are brought to the job, interfering with their production, their relationship to others on the job, and with their health. The length of absence from work depends on many variables, such as personality structure, environmental stresses on and off the job, motivations for health and illness, secondary gains, severity of the anxiety, etc. I try to keep these people working because I know that the regular routine of the day's living and the day's working is better for them than idleness and preoccupation with self at home. Psychotherapy should be continued during this time. I feel that people with mild and moderate anxiety reactions would be better off immediately and in the long run to stay on the job. They will not like us at once for insisting on this method of therapy, but they will ultimately be stronger to deal by themselves with the realities of life. If, in individual cases, persons with mild or moderate anxieties simply cannot work because of a poor personality structure or poor motivation, then their time off should certainly be minimal — a few days to 1 to 2 weeks. Unfortunately, the community physicians in many instances may be obstacles for us to keep these people on the job or to return them to work soon. The advice is, as you know, too often given to take a few weeks' rest in Florida or California. Experience teaches us that these people are usually no better and may be worse for so doing. Occupational physicians can help these people find the causes of their anxiety by being permissive, by adopting a listening attitude, by developing two big ears and one small mouth, and by encouraging them to talk or to ventilate about themselves on and off the job. A half-hour once or twice or a few times will in most instances be enough to help them to feel much better, to understand themselves a little better and to stay on the job. Brief psychotherapy certainly has been successful during World War II and the Korean conflict. I might say that it has been eminently successful in our hands in industry. You may say that you do not have the time to sit for a half-hour once or twice or thrice with a patient. But, how can you afford not to spend this time when one figures up the amount of 5 minutes or 10 minutes that many of these repeaters with anxiety state spend in the dispensary and in the doctors' offices. This total time is much more than if more time were given only a few times. The results are usually much more satisfactory if more time is spent with them initially. The costs of absenteeism to the plant will be markedly reduced and the employee will be feeling much better and grateful to you for "having given him your attention." It is true that deep insight therapy may not be achieved but brief psychotherapy by you will give them sufficient superficial insight to live more comfortably. Employees with severe anxiety which render them physically helpless will be out about 4 to 12 weeks. Interviews with members of the family, with supervision, and with selected other persons have helped me to return these people to work sooner. Hospitalization may be necessary and should be shortened whenever possible.

Neurotic-Depressive Reaction

The neurotic-depressive reaction with its many sad and sometimes severe bodily complaints occurs often enough to give us concern. This reactive depression develops as a reaction to something in the environment. Employees with mild reactions can usually work through the depression providing psychotherapy is also obtained. Symptoms such as mild blueness or sadness, a reduction in interest in things, slight anorexia, some insomnia, a feeling of not being just right, etc. can be reduced by sympathetic interest, a listening attitude by the physician, and by a few of the supportive medicines. As a rule there is no retardation of thinking or of action in these cases. The moderate and severe depressions will usually be out of work 2 to 8 weeks, depending on the individual's makeup and the stresses of the situation. Once again, interviews with members of the family may help out in this situation.

Schizophrenic Reaction

Schizophrenic reactions may be acute or chronic. The employee who develops an acute, sudden schizophrenic reaction usually has no predisposing schizoid personality traits. The person usually becomes ill suddenly from some environmental stress, hallucinates actively, behaves oddly, may be suspicious, and usually recovers in 4 to 12 weeks with very few residuals. The schizophrenic scars that we have known to have developed in so-called dementia precox usually do not occur in this condition. With modern psychiatric therapies these patients may be back to work quite soon with no personality scars. This reaction may be associated with marked mood changes so that the term "schizo-affective reaction" is sometimes used.

Patients who develop the more chronic type of schizophrenic illness are out of work for many months. With present therapies even these persons can return to work although their efficiency may be reduced. Returning the psychotic patient to work is a procedure needing a team approach. The team should be made up of many people, but ideally it should be made up of the supervisor, the occupational physician, the family physician, the hospital psychiatrist, the visiting nurse of the company or the visiting nurse of the local Visiting Nurse Association, occupational therapists, and social workers.

Manic-Depressive Reaction

Manic-depressive reactions usually subside in about 1 to 4 months with modern therapy. Of course, these conditions are subject to reoccurrences. These people are usually very efficient workers when well. Enlightened supervision will want to do everything possible to help them to return to the job and to keep them on the job. If the patient does not recover in 6 to 9 months, then, of course, permanent and total disability should be considered. If supervision is enlightened, understanding and concerned about their people, then the employee might be able to return to work earlier because support will be available at the work place. An interested supervisor will spend more time with these people and this facilitates the readjustment of the employee back to work. The supervisor should speak to the employee's coworkers to prepare them for the employee's return from the mental hospital by advising them to treat the employee like a "normal" person and not to ask embarrassing or silly questions. If a depressed patient returns to work too soon and then experiences failure on the job, he is apt to have a recurrence of his depression. He needs much support on his return to the job from supervision, from the medical department, from the family doctor and from his relatives, and, of course, from his psychiatrist if he is seeing one.

The Paranoid Reaction

The employee with a paranoid reaction causes much grief for all of us. Whether or not the paranoid employee remains on the job depends, of course, on the focus of his paranoid delusion and on the severity of the paranoid delusion. If the source or focus of the paranoid delusion is off the job, then the employee may be able to work continuously, providing he does not become upset by references inadvertently to his delusional system. If, however, the paranoid delusions stem from on-the-job sources, then he may become so anxious and apprehensive and his behavior so difficult that he may have to take some time off from work. Experience has shown to me that, in many instances, supervisors and coworkers have adopted an effective, healthy and tolerant attitude to the employee with a paranoid reaction which enables him to remain on the job and in a rather comfortable state. Certainly I know that much time is consumed by supervision and by the medical department in handling a situation of this kind. It is my feeling that these people are far better off working providing their behavior does not interfere with production and with the emotional climate of the department. However, when behavior begins to deteriorate, then the paranoid employee should take some time off and receive some therapy in a hospital if necessary. Modern psychiatric therapies certainly have rendered many of these paranoid personalities capable of performing their usual work. In the mild or moderate paranoid reaction, they may be out of work from 4 to 8 weeks. In the severe paranoid reaction, of course, they may be out many months and some never return.

Involutional Reaction

The involutional reactions, especially the malancholias, cause absences of about 2 to 8 weeks. Modern therapies aid the return to work in a very short time. Psychotherapy should, of course, continue after work has been resumed. The many physical complaints that these people suffer from interfere markedly with their working capacity. If the depression is not too severe, then I feel that they should be urged to continue at work. However, we know that in the severe cases work is impossible and they must be hospitalized.

I have not been as dogmatic as you or I would like to have had me be. This is because we do not have all the answers. There are so many variables and so much individualization in psychiatric disorders that a rigid healing time for psychiatric disorders is impossible to formulate at this time.

All of us who have to deal with these neurologic and psychiatric problems in industry might be reminded from time to time of the age-old adage, "I am my brother's keeper."

REFERENCES

1. Collins, R. T.: Optimum time off from work for neurologic and psychiatric disabilities. Indust. Med. 25: (Sept.) pp. 408-412, 1956.

17. The Placement and Management of Employees with Psychiatric Disabilities

THE MANAGEMENT OF THE NEUROTIC AT WORK

ONCE THE PATIENT has accepted the idea that his symptoms are due to "nerves" or "emotions," the occupational physician should try to get the patient to see a physician who can carry on with psychotherapy. This may be the patient's family physician. If there is no family physician or the patient does not wish to see the family physician, the occupational physician might refer the patient to a psychiatrist or a psychiatric clinic. In those areas of the country where there are no psychiatric facilities the occupational physician may be able to carry on psychotherapy himself. The following points might be kept in mind in this regard, viz.:

1. *Take time* — plenty of time — 30 to 45 minutes at least for each interview. Time taken early will save time later.

2. One does not have to find an organic cause for every symptom — this will relieve the occupational physician of his anxiety.

3. Develop two big ears and one small mouth. From time to time ask pertinent questions such as why, who, when, where, what?

4. Be understanding — rather than sympathetic.

5. Keep reality and common sense in focus for the patient.

6. Remember that a patient will develop likes and dislikes for each physician — positive and negative relationships — or transferences. It explains why patients fail appointments, get angry at you, get well or worse suddenly, etc.

7. Dependency on the physician may develop and it will have to be gradually dissolved later. We use the dependency relationship as part of therapy, but it must be dissolved later on.

8. Be friendly, warm, and genuinely sincere.

9. Help the patient to gradually reaccept the responsibilities of the job, the home, and life in general — to face up to reality. Get him back to work as soon as possible. Work is good medicine — it is good therapy.

10. Don't get discouraged if you don't seem to get answers to the patient's problems in the first or second or third or fourth interviews. Keep on listening in subsequent interviews. Remember that bells will not ring, whistles will not toot, and lights will not flash when the cause of some of the patient's problems might be found. Sometimes the cause and the source of problems come very slowly.

THE MANAGEMENT OF THE PSYCHOPATH AT WORK

I deliberately use the term "psychopath" because most occupational physicians understand what this term means, viz., the irresponsible social misfit who is not neurotic, not psychotic, not mentally defective, and yet not normal. In the older terminology the term used to define this type of personality was constitutional psychopathic inferiority. This person is selfish, immature, egotistical, never profits by experience or punishment, never faces up to reality, lies consistently, follows no moral code, and is very disruptive in any society in which he lives. When supervision, industrial relations, or somebody else in the company complains about the employee who is a psychopath, the physician should remember these points, viz.:

1. One does not cure a psychopath — one might help him to modify his behavior, or alter his attitude if he wishes to have help. This would be done in order for the individual to live in society and not to disrupt the group in which he works and lives.

2. Let him talk — to ventilate his thoughts, his feelings, his attitudes, his philosophies, his gripes, his hostilities, etc. If he can develop a positive relationship to the occupational physician, the physician might be able to carry him along with a minimal of disruptive outbursts in the group in which he works.

3. Be honest, fair, and scrupulously sincere and understanding. Try to get him to see his responsibilities as a mature adult.

4. Don't let the supervisor in the department suffer too long with the problem of the psychopath.

5. Give him one or two chances to shape up to discipline of the department and if he doesn't, then administrative measures should be taken by his department.

6. These patients are very persuasive, confident and sure of themselves. They will tell a plausible story, but the physician should first check with other family members before believing everything the psychopath relates. This has to do also with checking with supervision of the department in which the psychopath works.

THE MANAGEMENT OF THE PSYCHOTIC AT WORK

When an employee becomes acutely disturbed at the work place, the occupational physician should take steps to see that the employee is admitted at once to a hospital for psychiatric care. In most communities, there are procedures whereby an emergency psychiatric patient can be legally admitted involuntarily for observation for a determinate number of days, without court commitment. The rehabilitation of a psychotic employee begins the day he becomes ill. The goal is vocational rehabilitation as a part of total rehabilitation. The supervisor, co-workers, dispensary nurse or company visiting nurse, company physician, and other interested workers at the work place should keep in touch with him through frequent visits. The policy of the company should be to welcome back to the job the employees who have been ill with a psychiatric illness and who can return to some kind of employment. There should be close liaison between the hospital psychiatrist and company physician relative to the return of a psychotic patient to work. Matters such as the following will have to be discussed, viz.: Where should the patient work? Old job or a new job — part time or full time — heavy work or light work? Alone or with people?, etc.

Many psychotic persons can work effectively in spite of their illness. Paranoid personalities can function well if their delusional system is not stimulated. Schizophrenics can work well if supervision understands the problems involved and the physician keeps in touch with the patients, supporting and reassuring them. Moderate and mild depressive patients can continue work with help. The following points might be kept in mind in managing the psychotic patient:

1. Many psychotics are not cured. They can learn to live with their beliefs, attitudes, and feelings and at the same time earn a living and live in society.

2. Let the paranoid employees visit with you occasionally to let them ventilate their feelings and ideas.

3. Don't argue with a paranoid employee about his ideas and feelings. You only get yourself and him upset.

4. Follow up with all the psychotic patients in your office. Support and reassure them.

5. Keep in touch with their families. When managing any psychiatric patient. one must spend much time with the families of these patients as they want guidance in caring for their sick relative. and also the physician may be able to pick up helpful points about his patient.

6. Don't let the supervisor suffer too long in trying to help your psychotic patient adjust to the job. Put him on sick leave again if he is not well enough yet to work or put him on another job that may be less demanding.

7. Before a psychotic patient comes back to work from the hospital the supervisor in the department should inform the co-workers that the return of the patient is imminent and he should warn them to treat the person as if he were a normal person. Nothing should be done or said to embarrass the patient who is coming back to work. If the supervisor handles this educational program satisfactorily, the person returning to work from a mental hospital will be welcomed and managed very well by the co-workers.

8. We hope that there will be better opportunities in the future for employment and reemployment of those persons who have had a mental illness. The President's Committee on the Employment of the Physically Handicapped has recently accepted this group of handicapped people into their promotional and educational programs throughout the nation. We look forward with hope to what this Committee might be able to do.

A few brief case histories might illustrate the point that psychotic people can work effectively on the job from time to time and especially when they are being followed by an occupational physician or a psychiatrist.

Case #1. A 47 year old colored married man had worked at the company for about five years when he became confused, disturbed, and heard voices telling him to do certain things. Following a stay in a mental hospital of a few weeks, with shock treatment, he returned to work and has been working for a year and a half at the present time. He is back at his old job which was that of a maintenance man, working the C trick or the midnight shift. He had returned to work for a few weeks before he began to realize that he was having much difficulty in sleeping because the voices would keep him awake. He would go to bed about nine o'clock in the morning and have much difficulty in sleeping during the daytime because the voices would tell him to do this and tell him to do that. He said to his supervisor that he was having trouble sleeping and this meant that he could not give the company his best services, and this was costing the company money. He asked the supervisor if he could see the company psychiatrist. At the present time I have been seeing this patient for about a year and a half at intervals of approximately six to eight weeks. I placed him on thorazine, 50 mg., four times a day and seconal, gr. $1\frac{1}{2}$ at bedtime. Throughout the past year and a half he has been getting more sleep because he has been calmer and more relaxed. At the present time he is taking one thorazine spansule of 150 mg. at 8 a.m. and 8 p.m., and he is taking $1\frac{1}{2}$ gr. nembutal when he goes to sleep at 9 a.m. He still says the voices keep him from going to sleep and at times wake him up, ordering him to do certain things. He has been very faithful in his visits to me and his work in his department is quite satisfactory.

Case #2. This is a 46 year old married man with three children, age 10, 14, and 15, who came to see me because he felt quite depressed, was having sleeping problems and not eating well. He was still working but saying that he was not doing the job that he should be doing. I had seen him previously at that plant in 1951 for a hypomanic episode and in 1956 for another hypomanic episode. At this time he is suffering from a moderate depression. Allowing him to ventilate his feelings about his job and about life in general he has been able to stay on the job and do a creditable job according to his supervision. I placed him on an antidepressant and a tranquilizer and he is doing very well at the present time. It appears that he will not have to be hospitalized for this attack. He still says that he is tired out most of the time and that he has to push himself. He is on work which is quite detailed and yet he feels that he is able to do it well.

Case #3. This is the case of a 58 year old married man with no children whom I have been seeing off and on at the plant for about eleven years. I saw him in 1949, in 1956, again in 1959, and again in 1960. In all of these episodes he has been depressed and paranoid. He has been able to work all of the time that he has been feeling depressed and suspicious, but I have been able to support him by allowing him to ventilate his feelings against certain people in the plant and outside of the plant. His supervisors say that they are trying to understand him and they have worked with him very well throughout the years. They understand that he is somewhat queer at times and says and does strange things but in general, they have accepted all of these things and have humored him and helped him along. Within the past two months he has become depressed, paranoid, and agitated again, and after seeing him for three times he felt much better and was able to go back to work. He seems to think that supervision picks on him every now and then and says that everything he does is wrong. A certain waiter in a certain restaurant where he eats his meals from time to time picks on him, according to the patient. There is close liaison between the medical department and his supervision from time to time. This man has been able to work consistently even though he has not been well on occasions.

DEPRESSION AND SUICIDE

The occupational physician will see a number of depressed patients in his daily work. He should be able to recognize a depression "when he sees one" because the management of a depressive patient is delicate and suicide is always possible. The following points should be remembered:

I. Between 1930-1960 an average of 17,000 suicides a year were reported in the United States.

II. Causes for suicides in males:

> ill health — 40%
> domestic affairs — 3%
> love affairs — 3%

III. Causes for suicides in females:

> ill health — 20%
> love affairs — 10%

IV. Who suicides? Mostly depressed people; however, others do, viz.: excited, confused, or delirious people, schizophrenics (usually catatonics and hebephrenics) hypochondriacs with delusions, people with exaggerated fears of insanity, nihilistic delusions, ideas of persecution and torture, and patients who have previously attempted suicide.

V. Why suicide?

  1. No one or nothing to love — or be attached to.

  2. A conflict — involving demands on world.

    a. His angry sense of deprivation.

    b. His guilt.

    c. He has not worked out an adequate balance between giving and taking, and between aggressive and creative strivings.

    d. A turning of ones aggressive drives on to oneself.

    e. Driven to suicide, through despair, by nagging relatives to:

      1. "Snap out of it."

      2. "Use some will power."

VI. Points about depression.

  1. Every depressed patient is potentially suicidal.

    a. All threats should be taken seriously.

    b. High suicide rate.

      1. Mild to moderate depression.

      2. Agitated depressions.

      3. As depressions lift.

    c. Low suicide rate.

      1. Profound depressions — too sluggish to suicide.

    2. Biologic signs of depression.
       a. Insomnia.
       b. Poor appetite.
       c. Sluggish bowel activity.
       d. Sad look.
       e. Depressed.
       f. Sluggish thinking.
       g. Sluggish motor activity — patients are slowed up.
    3. Physical complaints and symptoms often are first signs of a depression.
    4. Look for the following:
       a. Signs of reduced energy output.
       b. Changes in interest, loss of interest and drive.
       c. Changes in the way things appeal to patient.
       d. Failure to get usual sitimulation out of things — no bang out of life.
       e. Insomnia — early awakening at first, then, can't get to sleep, develops many worries and paces the floor — chain smokes and frets during night.
       f. Anorexia.
       g. Weight loss; gastrointestinal upsets; low calory, inadequate intake.
       h. Mood changes — they say they feel fine but careful questioning reveals:
           1. Discouragement.
           2. Disgust.
           3. Disappointment.
           4. Complaints of physical condition.
           5. Slow thinking.
           6. Self accusation.
           7. Feelings of unworthiness and guilt.
           8. Gloominess, down in the dumps, the blues.
           9. Decreased talking.
          10. Increased apprehension.
          11. Decreased initiative.
          12. Sits all day and mopes.
          13. Mood swings.

i. Types.
  1. Reactive or situational depressions.
  2. Melancholias, mostly of involutional period.
  3. Manic-depressive depressions — spontaneous, recurring.
  4. Agitated depressions.
j. Severity.
  1. Benign.
    a. Patient seems not too hopeless.
    b. No overt attempt at suicide.
    c. No threats of suicide.
    d. Biologic signs of depression are minimal.
    e. Out patient treatment usually is satisfactory.
  2. Malignant.
    a. Threats or/and attempts at suicide.
    b. Patient has above biologic signs of depression.
    c. Should be hospitalized.
k. Remarks.
  1. Consult relatives for a clearer history.
  2. The physician should watch patient during therapy sessions for signs of hopefulness or hopelessness. If hopelessness seems to be developing, better check with the relatives and advise hospitalization.
  3. Early detection of depression is vital.
  4. Early referral for psychiatric help if this is available.
  5. Relationship between depression and accident proneness does exist.
  6. Watch the prescription writing of barbiturates.
    a. Keep number of pills to a minimum per prescription.
    b. No refills.
  7. Record all suicidal attempts.

18.   *Psychiatry in Occupational Compensation Injuries*

THE OCCUPATIONAL PHYSICIAN should realize that sooner or later he will be met with emotional problems that seem to arise from an injury on the job. The most common injuries to give rise to emotional components are back and head injuries. Whether one uses the term "traumatic neurosis" or any other label, the fact remains that a series of signs and symptoms develops in many patients following an injury to the body. One also runs up against the term "compensation neurosis" from time to time. This stems from the belief of many people that the individual who is injured from some type of work has as his goal the recovery of money or a secondary gain. And, as has been said in *The Mind of the Injured Man, by Dr. Fetterman*,[1] "The outlook for the recovery of an injury on the football field is a good deal better than that of an injury sustained when at work through slipping on a slippery stairway." As Dr. Foster Kennedy remarked in this same book, "For, as I once defined a 'compensation neurosis' to a truculent attorney who begged for punishment: It is a state of mind born out of fear, kept alive by hope — and stimulated by lawyers."

The author does not wish to go into any long and detailed accounts of the various injuries of the body and some of the consequent emotional and mental symptoms which may occur case by case. He wishes only to mention a few of the more salient facts which have come out of the study of the injured worker. These facts may aid the occupational physician of today to first recognize the possibility of the existence of the emotional and mental complications of an injury; and second, to attempt to understand why they have developed, in the light of modern day understanding of the human personality; and third, what to do about it:

1. Following every injury there is always the possibility that emotional and mental states may develop.

2. The symptoms and signs directly related to the accident may begin to recede as time goes on, but instead of completely disappearing, they may be reinforced by newer symptoms which develop. These

are based upon attitudes, ideas, thoughts and feelings that have developed in the time space following the accident.

3. The mental balance of the injured worker is always upset by an accident of any kind to any part of the body. It is always a threat, even a partial threat, to his life. The smooth functioning of his body has been disturbed and he reacts with many symptoms and signs.

4. The entire viewpoint of the individual may shift from work to worry and from the normal effort to introspection, as Dr. Fetterman has so aptly stated.

5. Dr. Fetterman continues, "There may follow the succession of emotional reactions, including self pity, the seeking of sympathy, and perhaps the quest for compensation against the party whom the injured party blames for the accident."

6. We know that there are a number of accidents that occur in which the individual who suffered the accident has been more or less unconsciously waiting for the accident to happen. The term "accident-prone" is not to be used in this regard. In fact, the term "accident-prone" is not being used as frequently and as strongly as it used to be. These people seem to welcome an accident as a relief from their trials and tribulations of their harrassed life. In this way, they seem to be honorably discharged from the battle of life and can now get some rest for a while. This situation is somewhat similar to the infantry man in combat who welcomes a wound so that he can be relieved of the necessity of fighting in the combat zone and can go back under an honorable diagnosis. In this way, he saves his face and saves his life. This is somewhat similar to these people who are injured on the job. One might say that they have lived a neurotic life all of their lives and have been functioning at a lower standard of performance.

7. The occupational physician should make sure as soon after the injury as possible that an examination is made of the injury, as assessment is made, and a course of action outlined for therapy. Most of these injured people will be referred to outside physicians who then direct the course of therapy.

8. In many of these cases, it is not only the injured worker who is involved, but also friends, relatives, lawyers, other physicians, etc.

9. The most common form of a psychiatric condition to follow an accident is the so-called "traumatic neurosis."

10. Traumatic neurosis may follow an insignificant injury or a

more serious injury. A period of unconsciousness may or may not have occurred following the injury.

11. The incubation period for the development of traumatic neurosis varies from a few days or weeks to, at times, months.

12. In these cases, usually there is no demonstrable evidence of any injury to the nervous system.

13. Industrial accidents produce most of these cases. However, they have occurred in other types of accidents such as occur in automobile accidents, railroad accidents, injuries sustained during combat, etc. Proximity to an explosion in war time and civilian life has been known to produce the traumatic neurosis in the absence of any organic involvement of the nervous system.

14. Traumatic neurosis most commonly follows injuries to the head.

15. The two main symptoms of a traumatic neurosis following a head injury are headache and dizziness. There may be other symptoms such as weakness, irritability, crying spells, shaking spells, apathy, noises in the head, ringing in the ears, generalized tremors, insomnia, poor concentration, poor memory, feelings of faintness, shortness of breath, etc. Occasionally one sees many hysterical symptoms, such as bizarre gait, staggering gait, hesitant gait, odd positionings of the body, many awkward bizarre movements of the body when the patient takes off or puts on his clothes or attempts to perform any of the neurologic tests, splinting of the body in getting up from a chair or laying down on a bed, etc.

16. Because of the fact that so many of the cases of traumatic neurosis occur in industrial accidents and litigation of compensation cases, some physicians feel that there is no such entity as a traumatic neurosis, but only a compensation neurosis. This is because of the theory that these cases represent an actual or possible gain to the individual.

17. As Wechsler states in the chapter on "Trauma and the Nervous System" in his *Textbook on Clinical Neurology*,[2] ed. 8:

If one excludes from this group cases fostered by poor management on the part of physicians, bad advice on the part of lawyers, and true malingerers, there still remains a large class which cannot be easily dismissed simply as a litigation neurosis or hysterics. Among the last, one can only include those individuals who find in illness an escape from unconscious difficulty. The trauma in these cases serves as the precipitating cause of conversion hysterical symptoms. The mechanism being exactly that of all other hysterias. To escape the drudgery of existence, the grinding monotony of industrial life, family conflicts, or what not, the individual unconsciously makes use of the trauma. That he thereby gives up the living wage for the mere pittance of compensation is no sound argument, because the unconscious gain may more than outweigh the money loss. Nevertheless, the trauma stands in definite relation to the illness in an individual who had a neurotic personality or character make-up.

18. Some investigators feel that there are minute changes in the nervous system, such as are found in the concussion of the brain, and they have introduced the term "traumatic encephalitis or encephalopathy."

19. At times, patients who have had industrial accidents will have repetitive nightmares in which they relive the accident. The accident has represented a serious threat to the ego, as I have stated above.

20. Most traumatic neuroses have a bad prognosis.

21. No matter what kind of treatment or series of treatments are provided for the patient, they do not seem to get well until some kind of a settlement is made.

As Wechsler states about these cases,

A number of patients continue to have marked symptoms until they have received full and ample compensation, and no amount of treatment is of any avail. Those come dangerously near the malingering class. It would seem advisable to make immediate financial settlement and thereby remove all economic incentive to further sickness. Such settlement would have favorable influence even on cases which come under the heading of traumatic neurosis. In most instances, a just and fair appraisal can be made within a few weeks of the accident. Errors of judgement are hardly likely in more than 10% of cases, and those could be made subject to review after six months or a year.

Some examples of cases with injuries are as follows:

1. A married woman, age 55, was walking by the ladies rest room when a cleaning man asked her if she would check the room to see if there was anybody inside, as he would like to clean it. She went into the ladies room and slipped on a cake of soap on the floor. She bruised her right elbow, but there were no observable cuts to the elbow or to any part of the body. She went to her family doctor who x-rayed it and found no broken bones, and said that it was only a bruise and would only take a few days to heal. However, the pain did not recede and the patient stated that she could

not move her elbow and insisted on keeping it in a hyperflexed position with the upper arm close to the chest. Weeks went by, and she stated that she could not move her elbow at all, and that the pain was severe in the elbow and in the shoulder. Shortly, she stated that she could not move the wrist or the fingers. She held her wrist in a hyperflexed position with all of her fingers hyperflexed into the palm of the hand. As months went by and she visited doctor after doctor, the symptoms remained and so did the disability. Repeated x-ray examinations and clinical examinations by orthopedic physicians and surgeons, could find no organic reason for the continued disability. Her attorney, whom she had procured shortly after the accident because she felt that she was not given a fair deal by the company or her family doctor, suggested a psychiatric examination. The psychiatrist felt that this was a case of conversion hysteria indirectly related to the accident. The patient was most resistive to psychiatric investigation, but enough facts were learned to realize that there had been much difficulty between herself and her husband and she was forced to work. She resented this bitterly. Ultimately, following psychiatric investigation in a psychiatric hospital, she saw more doctors, and by this time the palm of the hand was becoming calloused and the fingers had become practically immovable. The fingers and fingernails were digging into the flesh of the palm of the right hand. Ultimately, some surgeon felt that some plastic operation might be necessary in order to relieve the pressure in the palm of her hand, and so this was done. She was seen by another psychiatrist who verified the diagnosis of the first psychiatrist and suggested that no more operations be performed. Up to a recent date the patient's right arm was still completely useless and she had a claw hand. No settlement has been made by the insurance company as of this date, after five years of disability.

2. The next case involves a businessman who was walking home from work when an automobile ran onto the sidewalk and forced him up against the wall. One of the fenders grazed him slightly but there were no cuts on the body and only a few scratches on the skin of one leg. He was shaken up temporarily but recovered immediately and continued walking home. Because of this incident, he was much later than usual in arriving home and his wife was quite concerned. On seeing him in the home, she asked him what happened and he told her what had just transpired. She said that he looked pale and weak and that he should go immediately to bed and rest as he probably had shock. So he went to bed and actually remained in bed until he died four weeks later from pneumonia. His wife and other members of the family and relatives and friends insisted that he stay in bed although the physician said that there was nothing organically wrong with him and that he should get up and move about and get back to work. However, he remained in bed, was fed in bed and treated as a

very sick person by his wife and relatives. He developed a conversion hysterical paralysis of both legs and soon of both arms. He had many somatic complaints and ultimately developed pneumonia and died. As I recall the case, the compensation case was settled in favor of the deceased patient. The judge in the case ruled that it was unfortunate that the driver of the motor car had struck a suggestible person.

3. The next patient involves a housewife who was cleaning her bedroom. While stooping over to dust the floor, she raised up and struck the top of her head on the corner of the dresser in the bedroom. She was temporarily dazed, had a slight sore spot on the top of her head, and after making sure that there was no cut, she continued to work. However, about four hours later she noticed a numbness in the left side of the head. The next day she noticed numbness around the left ear and the left side of the face. Two days following the accident she had numbness of the left shoulder and left arm. Because she had seen a certain neuropsychiatrist many years before for a mild anxiety state secondary to some family difficulties, she sought out the services again of the same neuropsychiatrist. After taking the history and performing the neurologic examination, he assured her that there was nothing organically wrong with her. She stated that she was very surprised that there wasn't anything found. She could not understand why she had all this numbness. Further investigation of her case found that nine months prior to this household accident her father-in-law died. She was about three months pregnant at the time and had much difficulty with early months of pregnancy. During the rest of her pregnancy, she had continual problems with her husband who, although a good provider, never spent much time at home. Her delivery was a difficult one. The newborn baby, the trouble with her husband, the loss of her father, plus the care of four other children and her invalid mother proved too much for her. The minor blow on the head opened the floodgates, as it were, of all her troubles. Following conferences with her husband and with her, she recovered and the household was a healthier household afterwards.

REFERENCES

1. Fetterman, J.: The Mind of the Injured Man. Chicago, Industrial Medicine Book Company, 1943.
2. Wechsler, I.: A Textbook of Clinical Neurology, ed. 8. Philadelphia, W. B. Saunders Co., 1958.

19. Special Considerations in Occupational Psychiatry

THE TROUBLED EMPLOYEE often becomes a medical problem to the occupational physician. The following statement is taken from an article entitled *The Troubled Employee* by Milton Golin in the Journal of the American Medical Association:[1]

In one day several years ago, five employees of a large East Coast industrial firm went to supervisors to complain about their jobs: Schedules were too difficult. Co-workers were intolerable. Office equipment was no good. Other departments were uncooperative. There was too much noise — or glare — or heat — or cold. Because they also complained of backache, headache, and abdominal pain, they were referred to the plant medical office. There, a company physician who happened to be a psychiatrist listened to their gripes and relieved their hurts. He also found that only one complaint could be traced to actual work conditions. These were the true causes of the other four:

A stenographer whose boy friend had stalled her for a long time had become panicky at the thought of losing him.

An account executive was afraid he would inherit the heart disease that killed his father, and the paranoid tendencies showing in his mother.

A young salesman was ashamed that he could not make up his mind about the two girls who were in love with him.

A foreman was sick with the feeling that he was to blame for his wife's depression, which led her to threaten the lives of their two children.

How much business did the salesman lose that day? What major blunder crept into the steno's work? Where did the account executive fail to make an important decision? How many workers reacted in what way to the mood of their guilt-laden foreman? These may be questions for the economist, the sociologist, the administrator. But they also are questions for the family doctor. The troubles of these four employees, as of thousands more weighed down with anxieties, concern the entire medical profession because both personal and public health are at stake on a nation-wide scale.

Our experience has shown that 25 per cent of workers have personality disorders showing up in:

1. Absenteeism
2. Accidents

3. Alcoholism
4. Illness
5. Job dissatisfaction
6. Trouble with co-workers and supervisors
Of these, I shall discuss, Absenteeism, Accidents and Alcoholism.

ABSENTEEISM

Absenteeism is a continuing problem for everyone in places of work. The supervisor, the personnel man and the occupational physician are usually involved in cases of absenteeism. More and more statistics are showing that emotional problems of workers produce a large percentage of the absentee problem. The important topic of emotional disorders in the lives of the workers has consumed many hours of conferences, work shop sessions, lectures, and wherever people meet who have to deal with the health problems of these workers. It would seem that every program which deals with occupational medicine or the total health of the worker has some topic on the program which has to do with the emotional health of the individual worker and the effect of emotional disorders of the worker, on the wife of the worker, the company involved, and of production. In recent years, since those people who deal with the problem at places of work have become more sophisticated about the ever-present problem of emotional disorders, they have become more aware of the universality and diversity of emotional problems. Also, in the recent years since the family doctor and the community physician have become more aware of the importance of defining more accurately the reason for the absence of the employee from work, better diagnostic formulations are being made. In this way, more and more frank diagnosis of emotional conditions are appearing on the report of the family doctors. Heretofore, the reasons for the absence of the employees had usually been stated in physical terms. Many of these terms were vague conditions such as low blood pressure, anemia, tiredness, exhaustion, nervous breakdown, weakness, etc. Most of the time these diagnostic labels masked a real psychiatric problem. The reporting physicians have discovered that, by accurately labeling the reason for the absence of their patient, they do not adversely affect the job of the worker and, in fact, enhance his early return to work. Only by accurate diagnosis can the occupational physician understand the real problem, investigate the problem, and try to arrive at a solution to the problem, whether the problem be on-the-job or off-the-job. He, of course, would be working in concert with the family physician. The occupational physician should keep in constant contact with the family physician in the hope that the patient will receive adequate care and, if necessary, psychiatric care. This procedure is, of course, a delicate one, because the family physician feels that he is in command of the case and many times does not brook any interference from any other physician. The success of this procedure lies in how deftly the occupational physician has built up an atmosphere of good will and of trust with the family physician. There are many companies whose medical departments have done this over the course of many years.

Occupational physicians should keep in mind that emotional factors are practically always present to some degree in each of their patients. If there is a diagnosable physical condition present, emotional problems will usually be present to a lesser or a greater degree. In many cases, the convalescence of these patients from their medical or surgical illness will be delayed because of emotional reasons. The astute occupational physician will constantly have his ear tuned to the possibility of the presence of these emotional factors. A few simple questions directed at the job life of the individual and his off-the-job life will usually divulge some of the causes for the emotional problems. If the physician feels that the convalescence does not seem to be going along as it usually does in a particular condition, the physician certainly should begin to make inquiries as to other possible reasons for the delay in the convalescence. Such questions as "How are things going at home? How are the children? How is your wife these days? How are things between you and your wife? Where do you live? What kind of a home do you have? Are you having any financial problem? Are you having any problems on the job that are upsetting you? Do you have any fears about coming back to work? How do you get along with your supervisor?" are all simple questions which usually bring out some problem which is near the surface. Once these problems are out, the occupational physician might be able to do something about them. If the cause of the emotional problem seems to be a job situation, then a frank and open discussion of the problem certainly is in order. It is usually not possible to change jobs, but certainly if it seems advisable after consultation with the personnel department and the supervisor this might be effected.

We must bear in mind also that, next to the common cold, emotional problems are the most frequent cause of absenteeism from work. Most of the people whom we see at work are ordinary people with troubles. There have been many conferences held throughout the country on "the troubled worker." The most common symptom which is found in these troubled workers is anxiety. This anxiety is usually due to problems, stresses and strains which have arisen in the life of the individual, either on or off the job. They may be so minimal that one usually does rot consider them as true and pure psychiatric cases. Nevertheless, they are people who are having difficulties in solving the problems of life. Some of these people will turn out to be inadequate and ineffectual people. They have been this way since birth and probably will always continue to be so. The best thing we can do for them is support them, reassure them and carry them along. At times, their inadequacy is so great that they cannot be tolerated at work any longer. This usually occurs when these inadequate people reach the menopausal age or the sixth and seventh decades when aging begins to take its toll. If these people cannot work any longer and they are holding up production schedules, they probably should be retired from the company.

Persons with anxiety are better off working than not working, unless their anxiety is so great that their behavior is paralyzed. Work is good medicine for these people, as it channels off much energy into useful occupations. Too many times persons with anxiety are advised by their physicians to go south to Florida, or to Arizona, or to the mountains for a rest. These persons usually arrive back from the "rest" worse than when they left. They took their problems and their anxieties with them and they brought them back with them.

The point I wish to make is that, by and large, people with anxieties, mild depressions, fears, and the ordinary day to day worries should be urged to continue work if at all possible. Whenever the occupational physician has a problem of continued absenteeism on his hands, he should remember that there is undoubtedly an emotional factor involved. It is up to the occupational physician to try to ferret them out so that they can be dealt with in the open. This will reduce absenteeism, strengthen the patient in that it will help him to deal with his own problems in a mature fashion, and also it will aid the company and the employee from a purely practical viewpoint.

ACCIDENTS

Ever since safety departments were first organized many years ago, the aim has been to make the place of work as safe as possible. This has been done by instituting policies, procedures, safe practices and making the machines as safe as possible. Safety engineers have been concerned for some time with these factors. However, at the present time, the safety education program has reached the point of diminishing return unless the factor of human failure is considered, according to one superintendent of a safety department of a large company. As it has been said, "Accidents do not happen 'by accident.' " Most accidents are preventable and are caused by many factors. As Ross states in his chapter on accidents and their sequellae in his book, *Practical Psychiatry for Industrial Physicians.*[2]

We are not concerned here with problems of mechanical failure in the production of injuries. These aspects are being given adequate attention by engineers. They are outside the scope of the industrial physician, except for his concern that his plant safety program is including attention to mechanical failure by the engineers. We are concerned with problems of the human failure in the production of injuries. Granted that attention to mechanical failure should not be relaxed, human failure has not received attention in proportion to its contribution to injuries as mechanical failure has.

Today, safety engineers are aware that the problem of human failure is an important and difficult one. They are asking for help in this field of human behavior. Occupational physicians should be aware of the role of emotions and personality in the causation of accidents. The following points should be remembered in relation to the correlation between occupational accidents and human failure (modified from Ross[2]):

1. The prevention of human failure leading to accidental injuries is within the province of the occupational physician and is an important area for his collaboration with others in his company.

2. Some kind of case-finding technique for attacking the accident problem, from both a mechanical and a personal viewpoint should be set up by the occupational physician and others in his company.

3. Some kind of a treatment program should be considered by occupational physicians in order to produce a reduction in the accident rate.

4. Schulzinger[3] has recently written a book entitled "The Accident Syndrome." He points out that there is probably no accident-prone personality type, but that people move in and out of the accident-prone group, depending on the stresses and strains of life at the moment.

5. Nevertheless the concept of accident-proneness is still under scrutiny, ever since Dunbar discovered "by accident" that there were certain personality traits in people who had multiple injuries.

6. Dunbar found that these traits consisted of the following: decisiveness, impulsiveness, concentrating on immediate pleasures and satisfactions, acting on the spur of the moment, strict family upbringing, resentment against authority, tending to rebel against external authority, and against their own reason and self control.

7. Unconscious motivation is present in a high percentage of accidents, including revenge against authority, combined with self punishment for guilt about anger against authority.

8. The age of 21 seems to be the peak age of all accidents. However, Ross quotes Schulzinger as saying that findings have shown that repeated accidents reach a peak in children between the ages of 5 and 9 years. As Ross states, these are ages when conflicts with authority outside and within the family are particularly intense.

9. Accident prevention is part of general mental health, involving concern for the early treatment for prevention of emotional disorder beginning with children and parents. In the occupational setting, it is tied up with the total human relations efforts.

10. One consultant in occupational psychiatry has suggested the following procedures on accident cases. (a) With the first accident for any worker, check the mechanical and environmental factors. (b) With the second accident, check the human factors by group consultation. (c) With the third accident, arrange a psychiatric referral.

11. "Narrow escapes" from accidents should also be considered in the same fashion as actual accidents. The emotional factors involved may be the same.

12. Hurry, worry and flurry have been sighted as important causes of accidental injuries, both at home and on the job.

13. Home accidents are caused just as much by emotional and personality factors as occupational injuries.

14. Occupational physicians should be familiar with the literature on this subject and should work with the safety department, with the supervisors, and with the industrial relations department in a keen effort to prevent accidents and to reduce them.

15. As Ross states, "Accidental injuries, narrow escapes and hazardous working conditions, however caused, constitute a type of emotional stress."

16. In any accidental injury causing disability, emotional factors are always present and should be looked for and evaluated. When convalescence from a physical disability is slower than usually anticipated, the occupational physician should be more diligent in looking for these emotional factors. A traumatic neurosis can develop very quickly and very early unless these emotional factors are looked for, discovered and resolved early in the course of the accidental injury.

18. Emotional factors can be missed when occupational diseases of physical origin are suspected among workers in hazardous occupations, and, as Ross states "even in the condition known as "Miners Nystagmus" emotional factors, including traumatic neurosis, have been found. Emotional factors have been found in respiratory disorders, also."

19. Ross states that occupational physicians, civilian physicians and surgeons need more awareness of individual and group reactions to gross stress, not only for the sporadic occurrence of such stresses in modern industrial life, but also for the possibilities of mass stress in case of atomic warfare.

To point up the above points, the author reprints his article "Are You Accident Prone?" published in *This Week* Magazine December 11, 1960.[4] This was written for a lay public primarily but occupational physicians and safety engineers have shown much interest in the ideas expressed.

A few years ago medical science believed that people, endowed with certain troublesome personality traits, were especially prone to accidents.

Today, we don't believe that any more. Longer observation has enabled researchers to make a surprising discovery: the small group of people who have most accidents is not a fixed group, but a shifting one, with new people constantly becoming accident prone and others getting over it.

Our recent studies have reached this important conclusion: anybody can become accident prone during periods of stress and strain. In addition, medical investigators agree on another startling conclusion: very few accidents happen entirely by accident.

Most accidents are unconsciously desired. We really seem to want an accident which will help us solve a difficult life situation. We may even develop the accident habit to help us solve (temporarily) our problems. Like the girl who couldn't make the payments on her car — somehow she ran into a concrete bridge abutment, which washed out the car and, since it was insured, her debt at the same time.

Or there was Joe, who gambled on the horses, owed money to everybody he knew, was constantly angry at his wife's request for house money. Joe injured his arm at the plant and was off the hook for many months, safe in the hospital from the temptations of his bookie and the pressures from his debtors and his wife.

And there was Mary, who was fed up with her parents' continual objections to her boy friend. She managed to break her leg at work, and spent several weeks in the hospital with her leg in a cast — which, of course, insured her of sympathy, attention and babying from her family.

Mary wanted sympathy.

No basic problems were solved by those accidents. But these very average people were not able to face their problems squarely and deal with them — so they became, for the time being at least, accident prone.

Researchers believe there is another group of people who have accidents because they have developed certain ideas of the inadequacy of their bodies and their behavior. They accept their ineptness as being part of themselves from birth, like having red hair or blue eyes. Often they feel that because Mother was quick as a flash or Father was clumsy they are doomed to repeat the same accident-causing patterns.

In fact, we know they can help themselves by becoming more aware of their body and its behavior. These people should carefully analyze how they use tools or drive a car or cross streets, correcting their faults as they see them.

A third group has been recognized as the hard core of accident repeaters. These persons are usually aggressive, impulsive, imprudent, cocky, selfish. They care very little for others, profit not at all from past experienecs, punishment or the remembrance of pain, and they have very little respect for rules and regulations.

Because accidents are so tragically important economically and medically, costing in 1959 over 91,000 lives and 13 billion dollars, many studies have been made of the factors involved. Here are some findings:

Young people are more liable to have accidents, especially the 18 to 22 year old group.

Normally adjusted adults have accidents at a low, even rate through the age of 50, and then the number decreases steadily.

The summer months seem to produce more accidents than winter.

Accidents often occur in chain fashion, with the emotional stress of one leading to another.

Not more than 15 per cent of accidents arise purely from chance. Nearly all are caused by human factors. One investigator lists them: aggression, anxiety, boredom, discontent, excitement, frustration, grief, guilt, hostility, fear, indecision, lonesomeness, obsessions, preoccupation and rashness.

HURRY! WORRY! FLURRY! Those three words sum up the chief reasons for most accidents. Train yourself to be aware when you are hurried, worried, or flurried — and then be on your guard.

SEVEN ACCIDENT STOPPERS

1. If you're worried or under some other emotional stress, be more alert and on your toes than usual — or you may find yourself flat on your back. Postpone hazardous jobs.

2. Fatigue slows your reflexes, makes you more easily distracted and less alert, shortens tempers. If you have to drive or work when overtired, stop, look, listen and rest often.

3. Consider whether you're easily distracted from what you are doing — at work, while driving or at play. If you are, start a campaign to train yourself to "keep your eye on the ball."

4. Are there any accident hazards at your home or on the job that you should clear up? Are your car's tires and steering gear in good shape?

5. When you start a day by banging your elbow, spilling the coffee or bawling out the kids at the breakfast table with very little provocation, the yellow caution light should automatically blink on in your mind. Take the alarm — this may be your accident day!

6. Be mature enough to ask somebody to point out the potentially dangerous mistakes you habitually make while working, driving or around the house.

7. If you do have an accident, investigate the cause, and profit by the experience.

ALCOHOLISM

Alcoholism in industry is an ever-present problem and contributes much to absenteeism, disruption of production schedules, of morale in the departments, and to the ill health of the individual employee. Up until about the fifth decade of this century, this problem was not discussed much openly in industry. There was much concealment of the drinker and his problems, by his co-workers and even by his supervision. People felt sorry for these people and tried to help out in covering up for them and doing extra work for them when they were out because of alcoholic excesses.

However, in 1947 the Consolidated Edison Company of New York. Inc. officially recognized chronic alcoholism as a medical condition and adopted a "company procedure on alcoholism" and, as Pfeffer states in his Monograph on Alcohol in Industry.[5] This decision was based on a policy of meeting the problem openly instead of perpetuating the outworn pretense that it did not exist. The aim of the procedure was threefold.

1. The early recognition of the employee with a drinking problem.

2. Rehabilitation of the employee, if possible.

3. The establishment of a consistent basis for termination of employment when attempted rehabilitation failed.

Briefly, the administration of the company procedure of the Consolidated Edison Company in regard to chronic alcoholism is as follows:

1. The foreman and supervisor have the responsibility for the recognition of the early signs of uncontrolled use of alcohol among men working under them.

2. It is not the responsibility of the medical department to discover alcoholics, but the industrial medical department does have a role to play in the early recognition of the drinking problem which is masquerading as a medical illness. The medical department has the responsibility for diagnosis and for supervision of medical rehabilitation.

3. A training program for supervisors and foremen is in continuous operation to instruct this group to the understanding of the objectives of the "Company Procedure on Alcoholism" and to assist them in recognizing the early signs of problem drinking.

4. At the company, it was recognized that the following signs are indicative of the early phase of a drinking problem and often characteristic of the alcoholic "hidden man."

a. Consistent tardiness or absence on Monday morning and frequent occurrences of leaving early on Friday afternoon.

b. Unexplained disappearance from an assigned post during a tour of duty.

c. Recurrent excuses for absence due to minor illnesses or too frequent off-duty accidents, particularly with assault as a factor.

d. Personality change in a previously good worker; such as arguments with others, recurrent mistakes for which he defends himself, minor accidents which he blames on others or on equipment, marked variation in mood, and disinterest in his work.

e. The basis of the "company procedure on alcoholism" is the use of a firm, judicious, probation policy. This has been coupled with an adequate medical facility for rehabilitation. Probation is tentatively set at one year, with the understanding that it is really for an indefinite period. Since the employee may be denied progression increases depending on his length of service during the period of probation, the company limits the probation for one year to provide an incentive for his rehabilitation and a reward for his efforts. It would be poor psychology to extend this period officially. However, any relapse after the one year period still brings the employee under immediate review by the panel, as described below.

Pfeffer then goes on to explain the steps in the operation of the "company procedure on alcoholism." Occupational physicians are urged to read his Monograph on Alcoholism in Industry for a more detailed discussion of this problem.

The following general points about alcoholism in industry might be noted:

1. Chronic alcoholism is a common medical condition.

2. It often masquerades under the guise of a medical illness, so the occupational physician must be ever alert to this possibility when a medical illness cannot be explained by usually acceptable etiologic agents.

3. As Pfeffer states:

Alcoholism is a chronic, progressive and addictive disease, characterized by a craving for alcohol and its effect — a subjective state of well-being. The onset of the disease is based initially on a complicated psychological disturbance and facilitated by social and cultural factors. Once excessive drinking has begun in a psychologically susceptible individual, a series of additional processes ensues: nutritional deficiency, addiction, involvement of various organs of systems, and progressive psychological impairment. On the basis of these processes there follows further serious pathology of the organism at all levels of integration, with the development of a multitude of characteristic complications: medical, neuropsychiatric, psychological, social and vocational. The natural course of the disease is usually a progressively downhill curve on which there may be superimposed exacerbations and remissions.

Alcoholism may also be defined in simple terms as drinking that brings about, for the drinker or the people around him, serious problems in physical, mental, family, social or economic areas.

From the point of view of industry, a limited but practical definition of a problem drinker is: "An individual whose repeated or continued overindulgence interferes with the efficient performance of his work assignment."

4. Psychological factors appear to be the most significant etiological agent of alcoholism in the present state of our knowledge, says Pfeffer.

5. If there is not any definitive company policy in regard to the problem of alcoholism in his company, the occupational physician would do well to urge the adoption of some definite policy by top management for the spotting, treatment and rehabilitation of these people.

6. Pfeffer mentions the following medical complications of alcoholism, namely: acute alcoholism, alcoholic coma, gastritis, hepatic disease, cardiovascular disorders, and skin manifestations. He mentions that the alcoholic is somewhat more prone to infections, head injuries and other traumata than is the nonalcoholic. The alcoholic frequently shows evidence of

multiple illnesses against which, because of general debility, he is often unable to muster adequate defense.

7. Pfeffer mentions the following neuropsychiatric complications of alcoholism:

    a. Peripheral neuropathy.
    b. Wernicke's syndrome.
    c. Nicotinic acid deficiency encephalopathy.
    d. Marchiafava's disease.
    e. Pathologic intoxication.
    f. Delirium tremors.
    g. Korsakoff's psychosis.
    h. Convulsive disorder.
    i. Acute hallucinosis.
    j. Alcoholic deterioration.
    k. Alcoholic paranoid state.

8. Briefly presented here, he summarizes the psychology of the alcoholic in these words:*

The alcoholic is typically found to be essentially an infantile, self-centered individual. The image of himself is one of either omnipotence or of being small and incompetent. He is impatient of delay, intolerant of frustration and impulsive. He is sensitive and easily offended. Personal relations are tenuous and difficult. The alcoholic tends to be self destructive and may be openly or insiduously provocative. There is, in treatment, the ever present possibility, too, of drinking and becoming worse. An interruption of treatment is common. Depressive and paranoid trends are usually evident, and one must be aware of the possibility of psychotic features.

The treatment of the alcoholic is very difficult and fraught with much frustration. Motivation for treatment and rehabilitation must be genuine and strong. The typical alcoholic will use the mechanism of denial of alcoholism very often, and this denial mechanism interferes with therapy and rehabilitation. As Pfeffer says:

In recent years interest has centered on the possibility of undoing denial and establishing positive motivation in the alcoholic before the whole gamut of the illness has been run, and before the phase of 'low bottom' has been reached. It is striking to see how, just since 1952, industry can be effective in assisting in undoing denials and establishing positive motivation in alcoholics. The result in most cases is real improvement for the alcoholic and an advantage for industry in keeping an invaluable employee.

----

*The reader is urged to read Chapter 4 of Pfeffer's Monograph which is entitled *The Psychology of Alcoholism* for a concise statement of the facts of this condition.

9. Positive motivation can often be secured by the combined use of pressure and offers for treatment at some alcoholic clinic. Placing the employee on probation, with the understanding that should further difficulties arise involving drinking, he will be fired, and also offering him help for his problems often helps the individual develop realistic positive motivations.

10. The occupational physician should realize that the restrictions or presures that are applied on the alcoholic are warranted by the actual behavior of the alcoholic. In industry there is not only work inefficiency, absenteeism, and damaging of materials, but, in some instances, endangering of lives.

11. Methods of treatment consist of individual psychotherapy, psychoanalysis, group psychotherapy, the use of Antabuse along with these various therapies, and Alcoholics Anonymous. The hospitalization of an alcoholic must be determined by the individual circumstances of each case. Pfeffer discusses the pros and cons of other medical approaches to the therapy of the alcoholic.

12. Besides the New York University Plan for the treatment of the chronic alcoholic, with which Consolidated Edison Company of New York and a number of other companies in the Metropolitan area have cooperated, there have been other industrial programs for alcoholism developed throughout the country. These programs vary in detail from company to company in regard to the setting for the treatment of the alcoholic, whether it is inside the company, or outside of the company in a community clinic, or whether it rests solely on the services of Alcoholics Anonymous. Various alterations of some of the programs already in use certainly can be set up in any company, large or small, which is interested in salvaging the assets of an alcoholic employee for the sake of the individual employee and of the company and the community.

There are, in addition to the problems I mentioned at the beginning of this chapter, several other special areas for consideration; among them, promotion depression, transfer neurosis, the executive, his personality and environment, the hourly paid worker, the continued employment of persons with a history of psychiatric problems, and the problem of the retiring worker. A brief discussion of each of these will follow here.

PROMOTION DEPRESSION

The following are the facts in regard to this condition:

1. A person often develops depression and anxiety when he is promoted to a position with greater responsibility and demand for more training, experience, and ability than the person has had.

2. This usually occurs because there was not enough consideration given to the personality make-up of the individual to be promoted, his goals in life, his training, his experience, his ability to handle people, etc. Often, the person promoted does not want to be promoted and has no desire to be promoted, but these feelings on his part have never been known by those who promote him.

3. The person promoted becomes tense, depressed, fearful, develops insomnia, irritability, digestive disturbances, tiredness, weakness, and other medical symptoms. He is usually absent from work during this period.

4. The occupational physician should be aware of the impact of a promotion on a person who develops symptoms of a medical or psychiatric nature. He should be asked what he thought about his promotion; how he looks upon it; is he satisfied with it; or does the new job keep him awake at night? Many times these people will state "I did not want to be promoted. I am perfectly happy where I am. I don't want any more responsibility, and furthermore, I'm afraid I can't do the job."

5. The feeling of insecurity in the new job is quite common in these people who have been promoted. The insecurity may be valid and based on lack of training and experience for the new job. On the other hand, often the insecurity is based on some long-standing personality factors.

6. Top management is often quite surprised that a person refuses a promotion and wonders what the trouble is with that person. Management ought to realize that there are people who do not want to be promoted beyond a certain point, and these wishes should be respected. As we used to say in the military service, *one often makes a lousy* officer out of a good soldier. This can be transferred into industry when we say one can make a very poor foreman out of a very good worker, simply by promoting him to the job of foreman.

7. The occupational physician should attempt to educate those who are responsible for promotions in the company to the existence of this type of person in the company. A better selection system for promotion should be instituted by those departments charged with the responsibility of training. A more thorough consideration of the feelings of the person to be promoted, and of the ideas of the individual in relation to promotion and his goals in the company, would certainly forestall many promotions which were not wanted in the first place. A thorough talk before a definite step has been made would prevent a great deal of misery on the part of the promoted employee and also would prevent much expenditure of time, effort and money on the part of the company when a promotion turned out to be sour.

TRANSFER NEUROSIS

Transfer neurosis refers to a state of mind in which the individual concerned is constantly asking to be transferred to another department.

These repeated requests for transfer to other departments are not based on job misplacement. They are usually based on a certain type of personality make-up. It is almost as if the individual is saying to himself "The grass is always greener on the other side of the fence." He will usually give many reasons for his request to be transferred to another department, among them the following: "My friends in the other department say it's much nicer working there." "The boss is better." "The work is nicer." "You'll not have to work so hard." Or, there will be many complaints about the working conditions, people, type of work, materials, etc., in his present department. These people usually turn out to be persons who have never been able to stay in one place for very long in their lives. They seem to want to wander from place to place and never seem to have the stamina or the courage to stay in one place and work out their problems. Naturally, some people are bound to be misplaced on jobs, and therefore each complaint about the job should be taken seriously and investigated thoroughly. However, when one sees an individual who is constantly asking for transfers, one must bear in mind the possibility that this individual belongs in this class of emotional conditions.

Many of these people turn out to be inadequate and ineffective people who have never faced up to the reality problems of life and to the daily problems of living. They always seem to be blaming their weaknesses and failures on external things, such as the vagaries of human nature in the people with whom they work, on the climate, on fate, on their bosses, on their parents, their wives or husbands, etc. If one succeeds, through repeated requests, in being transferred again and again, the administrative processes of the company become disrupted, the departments upset, and actually the individual himself is being weakened from an emotional viewpoint because he is not facing up to the fact that sometime in life he has to buckle down and adjust to the problems of life. These people will howl the loudest when, after a thorough investigation has been made of their complaints or grievances and they are found to be adequately placed in a job commensurate with their abilities, training and experience, they are told that they are not being transferred. However, if one is sure of one's ground and sticks to his guns, these people will learn to adjust to their present jobs and, in some instances, become more effective employees and stronger personalities. Somewhere in their lives they have never been disciplined to take life as it comes and to adjust to it. The real cause probably goes back to a combination of constitutional endowment and environmental factors, probably in the home. Occupational physicians should be aware of this possibility and should educate those in the personnel department to spot these people early in their occupational life.

THE EXECUTIVE: HIS PERSONALITY AND ENVIRONMENT

The executive at any level in any company occupies a key position in regard to the total health of his employees. This is so because so much of his time each day is spent with people on the job. A recent president of a national business organization stated that America's number one industrial problem today is not production but people. People are our unfinished business, he stated.

The executive has the responsibility of seeing that work is done through people. If the executive does not realize that we hire the whole man, and not just his hand, then he is in trouble with his company. If he does not have a concern for his employees as human beings who have the same wants and needs out of life as he does, the health of his employees and the health of his company is in jeopardy. Much has been written in business and medical periodicals and in the lay press about the executive and his health, and the effects of the executive's policies on his company. The reader may refer, if he wishes, to a selected list of such articles in the index of this monograph.

The following are some points which I would like to note in regard to this situation:

1. The occupational physician has a unique opportunity to discuss the emotional health and the personality functioning of the executive of his company when these executives come to him for their periodic health examinations. In the course of these examinations, he should investigate not only the physical side of the executive's life but also his mental, emotional and personality side. This can be done in a casual way as one is talking with him about his health experiences of the past year, about his leisure time activities, about his stresses and strains, his community responsibilities, etc.

2. The occupational physician can carry on a continuing educational program on an informal basis, not only through the medium of the annual periodic health examinations, but also throughout the year when he is meeting the executives in various places throughout the company. The occupational physician is then carrying on his duties as the health officer of the company.

3. The occupational physician might practice the following attitude

himself, and when necessary, remind his executive patients of the following philosophical attitude. This is a quotation from Charles Dickens' "A Christmas Carol": "But you were always a good man of business, Jacob" faltered Scrooge, who now began to apply this to himself. "Business!" cried the ghost, wringing it's hands again. "Mankind was my business; charity, mercy, forbearance, and benevolence were all my business. The dealings of my trade were but a drop of water in the comprehensive ocean of my business."

4. The occupational physician might remember the following points in regard to the executive personality and his environment: I make these points because in many companies the occupational physician still sees the executives for examinations and he can help the executive become a more effective leader. Psychosomatic symptoms could be a good excuse for the physician to get the executive to talk about himself.

a. Has the executive thought about his role and function as an executive?

b. Has he given much thought as to what the public thinks about the executive? Today when a person has reached the executive's rung of the ladder, many people think of him as being omniscient and having the answers to all kinds of questions.

c. What kind of life does the executive lead off the job, with his family, with his friends, etc.

d. Has the executive developed any plan of operation for his life, both on the job and off the job, so that he will have some kind of a balance of activity. Is he working too hard or playing too hard? How has he handled the many requests to serve on community committees, boards of directors, of the various community agencies and organizations? Has he learned how to say "No" to some of these requests? I know of one executive, who, when he became a Vice President, decided along with his wife that he would spend his off-the-job efforts in only two activities: his church and the Boy Scouts. He and his wife decided that they would live in an area of town where not many of the people who worked in his company lived. They decided not to fraternize socially with too many people from his company. He decided that he would not bring any work home at night or on weekends, but he would get into work at 7 in the morning and leave at 6 at night. It is true that he refused many of his friends in the community who were at the same level in the managements of other companies in the community, when they asked him to belong to this committee or that organization or to give speeches here and there. However, he has maintained his sanity and health to a remarkable degree. Many times, if the executive feels that he is not achieving status in his own organization, he will seek for status outside of his organization in community activities, and many times he will overdo the latter. This will not only undermine his own health, but also he will not be producing effectively for his own company.

5. Inquire of the executive as to his level of irritability. Does he lose his temper? Has he forgotten how to be kind, thoughtful, considerate; has he lost sight of his goals in life, of his values and of his honesty? Does he still have a sense of humor which might carry him through some of the stresses and strains of everyday life? Has he found himself acting somewhat mean, prideful, vain, selfish and callous at times? Is he taking sufficient vacations throughout the year, and if so, how does he spend his vacations?

6. Has the executive ever tried to appraise himself? Has he ever asked his wife to rate him as a person, or, for that matter, has he ever asked his employees to do the same?

7. What are the hobbies of the executive? Does he have some interests outside of work to which he can devote his time, energy and efforts, and forget his job? How has he balanced his life between his job and his hobbies, his recreation and his community responsibilities? I like to think of this in terms of the chair of life. This a homely example, but it is suitable for the purpose. The chair of life is like any other chair in that it has four legs. One leg can represent vocation; another leg can represent avocation or hobby; a third leg might represent family, friends, religion, art, music, literature, etc., and the fourth leg might represent recreation. It makes no difference how each individual assigns the various areas of his life to the legs. One individual might like to have the chair of life rest on religion. Now, if a man works too hard and too long, the leg representing his job or vocation will become to long. The chair will then be lopsided and so will be his life. If a man plays too hard, then the leg representing recreation will be too long and the chair will be lopsided and so will be his life. The idea is to balance these four areas so that the chair of life rests foursquare on the ground most of the time during one's life. It is true that at times one's life is temporarily unbalanced because of pressures, stresses, strains, etc. The idea is to keep your life in balance most of the time.

8. The occupational physician might ask the executives during the periodic health examination some questions about the following areas of his life: overweight, shortness of breath, rising blood pressure, headaches, tension, restlessness, insomnia, rising alcoholic quota, the noon martini, irritability, short temper, short concentration, dizziness.

9. The occupational physician can point out to the executive the importance of his role as a father and a husband. Too many husbands and fathers neglect this role to the exclusion of their business. Does the executive recognize the needs and wants of his wife? Does he have adequate communication with her, or is she left to make household decisions herself

because the husband doesn't care to communicate with her? Does he give his wife sufficient attention, affection and praise? The wife probably once had a job also, as the husband does now. Has the executive ever asked himself what satisfaction his wife derives from her present job? Does the executive pay enough attention to his children? Does he play with them? Does he work with them in the cellar at crafts? Does he play sports with them? I remember a man who, when I asked him what kind of a person his father was, told me that he never knew his father. His father was a salesman during the week, and on weekends, he played golf in the summer and bowled in the winter. Consequently, the son and mother grew up together, practically oblivious of the male in the house.

10. Does the executive appreciate the fact that he should have an outlet for his aggressive drives, for his angers, for his mads, for his pent-up emotions, his tensions? I am reminded at this juncture of a Saturday Evening Post cover of a few years ago, that illustrates this point. In the upper left hand corner, the boss was bawling out the husband. In the upper right hand corner, it showed the husband bawling out the wife. He had his finger through a hole in a sock and he was giving his wife what-for because of her negligence. In the lower left hand corner, it showed the wife bawling out the four year old son, and in the lower right hand corner it showed the son bawling out the family cat. This is an unhealthy chain of events which occurs in many families, but which is not good. The husband should have some kind of outlet where he can let off steam, rid himself of his tensions, emotions, etc. He should have a punching bag in the cellar, he should go on long hikes or go fishing or hunting, he should play golf, pound the piano, etc. I know of a man who gets a great deal of delight in playing golf, because every time he whacks the golf ball he sees his boss's face mirrored there. I suppose that one might say that a person should always express himself emotionally but control his behavior. One should always express himself emotionally, but should not hurt people, animals or furniture.

11. Is the executive pretty well in control of his hostilities? How does he handle them? What about grievances? Can he forgive? How about his patience and his tolerance for the mistakes of others?

12. Does he have "briefcaseitis"? That is, does he take his briefcase home, stuffed and crammed to the gills every night; or does he leave his briefcase in the office and take his work home in his head? Either is bad. The executive should so organize his life that this would be unnecessary.

13. What are the value systems of the executive? Has he developed any mature, adult values for himself?

14. Has the executive asked himself what he wants out of his job? Is he aware of the effects of his behavior, his thinking and his feelings on people at his own level, on people above him, and on the people below

him? Does he have adequate communication with his associates, his subordinates, and with his superiors?

15. What about his decision making? Is he finding it increasingly difficult as the years go on to make decisions? Is this a symptom of over-work, tension, worry, etc.? Does the executive blame his job, the people, and his wife for his own faults?

The executive or supervisor at any level, therefore, should be a mature adult with healthy emotions and mental outlook. As I have stated in an article entitled "We Hire the Whole Man."[6]

The executive must realize that people who deal with people should know something about people — their motivations, hopes, emotions, personality make-up, and weaknesses. An employee brings to work years and years of some kind of personality development. Developed and molded in the home, school, church, society, and business or industry, we are today what we have been. If we are to change ourselves to adapt ourselves better to today's challenges, we should realize that we change slowly, but only after we have understood how we developed in our formative years. Patterns of thinking, of feeling, of working, of relating ourselves to our fellow beings, have developed slowly and are altered slowly. But a good supervisor is patient. Intuitively he understands all of this and will patiently go about his job of effective supervision. The employee may be helped by his religious advisor or his physician in many cases, and they, with the supervisor, can form a team approach to help the employee on and off the job.

Occupational physicians today are reading that the executive does not seem to be any more prone to heart diseases, high blood pressure, strokes and nervous breakdowns than any of the other workers in American industry. Years ago, some articles were written which created quite a stir among the executive ranks. Some of these articles were entitled "Your Next Promotion Can Kill You,"[7] "Why Executives Die Young,"[8] "Our Men Are Killing Themselves,"[9] "Beating the Odds on Executive Mortality,"[10] "Must Executives Die Young?"[11] "Executive Crack-up,"[12] etc. It isn't work that makes us sick, but worry over work. Most executives enjoy the hard, long hours of intellectual work, with the inevitable tensions which accompany decision-making, policy formulation, conferences, etc.

Worry is one of mankind's most prevalent and most disastrous conditions. The surveys show that 40 per cent of the time we worry about future things which never happen. Thirty per cent of the time we worry about past things about which we can do nothing. Ten per cent of the time we worry about our health, 12 per cent of the time we worry about what people think of us, leaving only 8 per cent of our time to worry about the day's problems, and this is not nearly enough time! As the executive learns to do the best he can each day and let the chips fall where they may, if he follows a philosophy such as this and organizes his time properly, if he has a sense of humor, treats people decently and humanly, then he will have learned to organize himself properly so that he will take up each problem as it comes along. He will let tomorrow's problems develop and will handle them himself tomorrow in the best way he can.

THE HOURLY PAID WORKER

Whenever the occupational physician is dealing with an hourly paid worker, some of the following points might be remembered as an aid in the handling of each case. Some of these outlined points were gathered from the chapter on the hourly employee in the book *Mental Health in Industry*[13] by McLean and Taylor.

1. The hourly employee has problems peculiar to him by virtue of his role in industrial society.

2. His operations are related primarily, if not exclusively, to the production of a given industry, whether it is devoted to turning out materials, supplies or services.

3. Above the hourly employee are the first line of supervision and the entire hierarchy of management. Below him is the machine, the production, or the servicing process, or the customer.

4. In consequence of this, he makes few decisions in any direct or controlling form affecting other human beings as regards production or services. To be sure, he may exert an influence on his foreman and others within the industry, but not in any direct or explicit fashion, rather, in an informal manner. In short, he controls directly the productive process only.

5. In general, therefore, he is in a position of accepting control and direction from others in his day-to-day activities.

6. In this general setting we might very well expect that there would emerge feelings of resentment and envy of other people in the industrial hierarchy who, rightly or wrongly, exert a direct and controlling influence on the industrial process.

7. Management should recognize and handle these feelings, because how such feelings are recognized and dealt with are important to the mental health of the work group.

8. It is important to develop the historical background in the present

setting in which these emotional reactions of an hourly employee take place.

9. The union as an institution in modern society has demonstrated its increasing growth and influence. Among the major reasons for this is that it mirrors and expresses the needs for security of its members.

10. Many grievances of the hourly employee ostensibly were related to the issue of wages, but really were not. Feelings of job insecurity, threats of management omnipotence, interpersonal resentment and feelings of rejection became displaced on this socially accepted group determined demand. Under the guise of demands for wage increases, are distorted and poorly defined feelings of insecurity. In the present era, issues concerning union recognition and general wage levels have fallen into patterns of annual or periodic adjustment. Unions are turning to other areas in an effort to satisfy their members more fully. Matters of health, guaranteed annual wage, pensions and the length of the work week are now coming sharply into focus. The union is striving to have its members become more actively interested in community affairs, education, and, at times, research.

11. Various types of conflicting loyalties may plague the hourly worker, may disrupt him greatly and may lead to impaired mental health. Examples of conflicting loyalties are as follows: the conflict between allegiance to the company and to the union, and the occasional conflict between the employee's own work group and the foreman. If the employee is oriented toward moving up to management's ranks, there is a conflict between himself and his work group, or within himself. So the position of the individual and his work group and his feelings about that social position are important to his mental health. There is also the problem of his acceptance or rejection by his own work group and, to some extent, by his supervisor. Of course, there will be personality differences — the dour nonconformist who keeps to himself is in a different situation from that of the easy going and well accepted group member. Different people see the work situation in different ways so that one man's needs are another man's poison. For most people, then, the informally developed loyalty pattern serves as a compromise between emotional needs and the social pressures of environment. Through the maintenance of this equilibrium, the hourly employee helps to preserve his state of mental health.

12. Automation has been variously described as a threat and as a promise to the hourly employee. Automation is spreading widely through many industries through improvements and technology. McLean and Taylor ask the question "How realistic is the so-called threat of automation? Are the current excitement and reaction to the imagined threat as clear cut as some would have us believe? Could the subject of automation rather be a target for the displacement of many other feelings of insecurity felt by the hourly employee?" There are those who feel that automation feeds

on an economy. So does a healthy work force. Jobs threatened by automation are replaced by new products, processes and ways of life. McClean
and Taylor seem to think that automation need not affect adversely the
mental health of the hourly employee. They mention that, as the machine
or electrical device displaces men, there is the threat, however, of the
omnipotence of the machine. There is a danger that, with the increasing
power of the machine, man himself may, in turn, gradually be treated more
and more as a machine and thereby be dehumanized. The increasingly
complex marvels of the electronic becomes awesome and God-like. This
danger is inherent in automation — that, in man's comparison of himself
with the omniscient machine, feelings of insignificance may arise.

13. With the hourly employee working shorter work weeks these days,
some of them will take on additional employment on the outside in order
to cut down leisure time. The economic gain in so doing must always be
remembered as an incentive for the second or third job. The occupational
physician must be aware of this, because the added work may be sapping
the strength of the employee. With more leisure time on his hands, the
employee does have a choice to make. The choice lies between recreation,
hobbies, or another job.

14. Boredom from too much leisure time may also impair mental health.
Some workers who, because of their personality or background, may not
be able to devise hobbies, pursuits, or recreation to take up the leisure,
may develop feelings of frustration, annoyance and exasperation.

15. The hourly paid employee may have difficulty in handling the relationships with his supervisor. This has to do with his handling of authority
situations; namely, his ability to accept instruction and guidance. If the
hourly paid employee fights against any method other than his own, or
if he resents direction and always seem to be at odds with his foreman, his
mental health is going to suffer and he is going to be quite unhappy. This
makes it imperative for the occupational physician to look into the setting
in which the employee works. The employee should be asked how he feels
about his job and his relationship to his supervisor, how he feels about
his machines and how he feels about getting along with other people in
his group. The occupational physician might be in a position to help the
supervisor understand some of these feelings of resentment or frustration.

16. The hourly paid worker likes to have a feeling of participation in
the work involved. Work as an activity in itself contains much in significance and value. If the employee does not have the feeling of the importance of work, his mental health will suffer. The worker likes to feel
that he is challenged on the job, and this helps his initiative and his ability
to accept the challenge. The more he feels that he is participating in the
productive process and the decision-making concerning the productive process, the greater will be his feeling of well-being.

THE EMPLOYMENT AND REEMPLOYMENT OF PERSONS WITH PSYCHIATRIC HISTORIES

It was not too many years ago when a person who had been in a mental hospital or even had seen a psychiatrist was turned down for a job or was refused reemployment following an emotional or mental illness. These attitudes are changing today, but there is still resistance to the entire idea of anybody with a mental illness ever being able to work again. Even in those companies which have adopted a policy that these people will be considered on the basis of their merit and ability, just as anyone else, the implementation of this policy runs into many obstacles at the hiring level. There are still too many individuals who do the hiring who have a very narrow outmoded concept of the person who has recovered or improved from a mental illness. Prejudices are still with them in regard to what they have known about or heard about the person with a mental illness. With the newer therapies in psychiatry being used more extensively, more and more people are improving to the point where they can return to their former jobs or can seek new employment. Many of these people can work and become once again functioning units in our society.

The occupational physician stands in a very good position to educate and orient those who develop policies of employment and reemployment and those who implement these policies at the hiring level in the personnel departments. The occupational physician can also, through his daily contacts with the first-line supervisors, help them to understand a person who is returning to work from an emotional or mental illness, as well as those who are working for the first time in a particular company following an emotional or mental upset. These individuals are fearful that such patients will "upset the apple cart" or "run berserk" or disturb the serenity of the department or office. If the selection and placement of each individual is carefully done following a program of working with the psychiatrist in the hospital or in the community and following his advice, then any untoward behavior on the part of these people will probably not occur.

The following points might be considered in this particular situation:

1. As emotional and mental illness become more understood by more people, more and more of these recovered psychiatric patients will be able to take new jobs or return to their old jobs in the various occupations.

2. The newer psychiatric therapies shorten the hospital stay and makes it possible for these people to resume their former ways of life earlier

than formerly including return to their work.

3. The occupational physician should work in close liaison with the psychiatrist in the mental hospital or in the community when one of his employees is ill with an emotional or mental upset. A definite program for dealing with an employee who has become ill and entered a mental hospital should be instituted from the time the employee enters the institution. This could be an informal program in which the supervisor, the company nurse (dispensary or visiting), the company physician and others interested in the situation could make frequent visits to the hospital when these visits are deemed to be all right by the attending psychiatrist. The occupational physician will then be able to advise the supervisor when the patient is ready to leave the hospital and when he is ready to resume work. Any recommendations as to how long the individual should work, what kind of work he should return to, and when he will be able to take up his full job with its attendant responsibilities can be translated to the supervisors.

4. The supervisor can be briefed by the occupational physician as to how he might prepare the other members of the department for the return of the person from the mental illness. In general, the employees should be advised to treat the returning employee as they would any other employee returning from any other illness. There should not be any unnecessary coddling or attention given to the person because this singles the individual out. The returning employee certainly wants to merge immediately into the group and not stand out significantly.

5. The occupational physician can also advise the supervisor that the returning employee may have some feelings of insecurity, that he may feel threatened by the job and by the responsibilities once more, and he may feel embarrassed or ashamed about the fact that he had *that* kind of an illness. A reassuring word now and then in a casual manner will usually help the individual gain support and confidence in himself.

6. The occupational physician should realize that there are no standards set up for the employment and reemployment of the person with mental illness. However, steps are being taken by the Joint Committee on Mental Health in Industry of the American Medical Association to set up such standards as soon as possible. It is hoped that these will be along functional and not diagnostic lines. In this way, the individual will be set as to what he can do and what he can't do.

7. In some state hospitals throughout the country, there has developed a system of workshops within the hospital buildings which resemble an ordinary industrial workshop. When patients are considered ready to once again return to work, they are placed in this in-hospital work setting. They are moved to the area in which they live and work. They are given jobs

commensurate with their abilities and their former occupations and are supervised as they would be in any other factory situation. They are paid the going rate within the community and gradually learn step by step and day by day to take up their work where they left off. There is, of course, a close liaison between the mental hospital and the industries of the community, and this works for the benefit of the individual who is recovering from a mental illness.

8. The President's Committee for Employment of the Physically Handicapped has recently adopted a resolution to promote more fully the employment and reemployment of those people who have had mental illness. This is a significant step forward. In implementing this resolution, a new committee was formed named The Committee on the Mentally Handicapped with the author as its first chairman. This committee encompasses the problems of the mentally restored and the mentally retarded. A first meeting has been held in Washington and plans for the work of the committee were discussed. The committee is also studying the possibility of removing the word "physically" from its title. This then would imply that all handicapped people would be considered in the work of the President's Committee. Several Governors' Committees have already dropped the word physically from their titles.

RETIREMENT AND PSYCHIATRIC PROBLEMS

When the working man has retired and he finds that he has no place to go in the morning, his mental health may be impaired. Many of these retired workers will come back to see their own occupational physician who has followed them for many years. Those who do return are usually those individuals who, because of their own personality make-up, and their neglect to broaden their interest into a number of different channels during their working years, now find themselves destitute of things to do. Depression and anxiety are very common. The worker who seems to have been married to his job now becomes depressed, fearful, frustrated and develops many physical symptoms, such as insomnia, restlessness, indigestion, weakness, easy fatiguability, etc. Their common plea to the physician seems to be the following: "The best medicine that you can give me, doctor, is to get me back to work at such and such a company." The depression may become so profound and so disabling that a psychiatrist may have to be called in and the patient may have to be hospitalized. If the depression and anxiety are mild and the individual is willing to attempt to do something for himself and become interested in some hobby or some other type of occupation, his symptoms will usually disappear. Motivation and initiative are so very important for these people.

This points up the wisdom of preparing individuals for retirement many years before actual retirement. Many companies today have annual or semi-annual reviews of the economic status of the individual at the time of retirement. Many other companies go further than that and go over not only the expected financial returns that the retiree can expect, but also begin to plan with him what he expects to do with his leisure time. It probably is never too early to start such a program in a formal way. Those individuals who, throughout their working lives have always been interested in community activities such as the Church, Red Cross, Chamber of Commerce, Service Club, and many other activities, will also have found much satisfaction and comfort in many different hobbies. Some even go into other kinds of occupations. There are many stories of retired engineers, physicists, chemists and others who have developed companies of their own and have become sub-contractors for the same companies for which they used to work. With older people staying healthier longer, the wisdom, training and experience of these elder statesmen of industry can very well be used to good advantage by society. Wise is the company that has a vigorous, dynamic, ongoing program for the education and orientation of their own employees looking forward to the time when they will not just retire, but will move into other fields of endeavor, satisfaction and challenge.

REFERENCES

1. Golin, M.: The troubled employee. J. A.M.A. (Nov.), 1959.
2. Ross, W.: Practical Psychiatry for Industrial Physicians. Springfield, Ill., Charles C Thomas, 1956.
3. Schulzinger, M. S.: The Accident Syndrome: The Genesis of Accidental Injury, A Clinical Approach. Springfield, Ill., Charles C Thomas, 1956.
4. Collins, R. T.: Are you accident prone? This Week Magazine, New York, United Newspapers Magazine Corporation, December 11, 1960.
5. Pfeffer, A. Z.: Alcoholism. New York and London, Grune & Stratton, 1958.
6. Collins, R. T.: We hire the whole man. The Rotarian, May, 1956.
7. Page, R. C.: Your next promotion can kill you. Look, April 7, 1953.
8. Bennett, R.: Why executives die young (abstract). The Management Review 41:270-271, May, 1952.
9. Lees, H.: Our men are killing themselves. Saturday Evening Post, January 28, 1956, p. 25.

10. Ratcliffe, J. D.: Beating the odds on executive mortality (abstract). The Management Review 42:66-67, February, 1953.
11. Must executives die young? (abstract). The Management Review 43:562-253 (Sept. 3), 1954.
12. Smith, R. A.: Executive crackup. Fortune 51:108-111 (May), 1955.
13. McLean, A. A., and Taylor, G. C: Mental Health in Industry, New York, Toronto and London, McGraw-Hill Book Company, Inc., 1958

ADDITIONAL REFERENCES

Occupational physicians may wish to have references to articles on psychiatry in industry and allied health subjects. The following is a list of suggested articles:

1. Baetjer, Anna M.: Women in Industry: Their Health and Efficiency. Philadelphia, W. B. Saunders, 1946.
2. Bishop, Jerry E.: Disturbed workers. Wall Street Journal, June 30, 1958.
3. Brody, Matthew: The dynamics of mental hygiene in industry. Indust. Med. 14:9, 760-773 (Sept.) 1945.
4. Dershimer, F. W.: Effective Discipline Promotes Mental Health Process, 6th Annual Meeting. American Academy Occupational Health. February, 1954, p. 36-40.
5. Eadie, G. A.: Practical methods for handling psychosomatic problems in industry. Indust. Med. 18: 369 (Sept.) 1949.
6. Felton, J. S.: Progressive industry and the worried employee. Mental Hygiene 37:545, 554 (Oct.) 1953.
7. Garrett, Annette: Interviewing (Its Principles and Methods). New York, Family Service Association of America, 1942.
8. Giberson, L. G.: Psychiatry in personnel work. Indust. Med. 12:164 (March) 1943.
9. Today's industrial psychiatry. J. Am. Med. Women's A. 2, No. 6, p. 280-281.
10. The technique of listening to the worried employee. Indust. Med. 9:414 (July) 1940.
11. Women in industry and the older worker. In Cameron, D. E., and Ross, H. G., Eds.: Human Behavior and Its Relation to Industry. Montreal, McGill, 1944, chapt. v.
12. Gordon, Gerald: Industrial psychiatry-five year plant experience. Indust. Med. 21:515, December 1952.
12a. Himler, L. E.: The place of psychiatry in industry. J. Michigan M. Soc. 49:75-78 (Jan.) 1950.
12b. Industry is the psychiatrist's new patient. Business Week. February 18, 1956, p. 56-59.
13. It's good business to know your men. National Institute of Mental Health of the U.S. Dept. of Health, Education and Welfare, Supt. of Documents, U.S. Government Printing Office, Washington, D.C.
14. Klemes, M. A., and Kallejian, V. J.: The group psychotherapist in industry: a preventive approach. Internat. J. Group Psychotherapy 5:91, 1955.
15. Kubie, L. S.: Psychiatry in industry. Ment. Hyg. 29:201 (April) 1945.

16. Larke, A. G.: Industrial psychiatry; aid to human relations? Duns Review, February 1954.
17. Laughlin, H. P., and Hall, M.: Psychiatry for executives: an experiment in the use of group analysis to improve relationships in an organization. Am. J. Psychiat. 107:493, 1951.
18. Levine, M.: Psychotherapy in Medical Practice. New York, Macmillan, 1946.
19. McAtee, Ott B.: The establishment and function of an industrial mental hygiene service. Am. J. Psychiat. 107: no. 8 (Feb.) 1951.
20. McLean, A.: Management discovers psychiatry. Think Magazine, International Business Machines, March 1959.
21. Menninger, W. C., and Levinson, H.: Human Understanding in Industry. Chicago, Science Research Associates, 1956 and 1957.
22. Psychiatry in industry, a key to better relations. Med. Advance 11: no. 4 (May-June) 1954.
23. The application of psychiatry to industry. Report No. 20, Group for the Advancedment of Psychiatry. New York, Mental Health Materials Center, July 1951.
24. Troubled people on the job. Committee on Occupational Psychiatry, American Psychiatric Association, New York, Mental Health Materials Center, 1959.
25. Vonachen, H. A.: Medicine in industry. J.A.M.A. 157:1592 (April 30) 1955.
26. Vonachen, H. A., Mittelmann, B., Kronenberg, M. H., Weider, A., and Wolff, H. G.: A comprehensive mental hygiene program at Caterpillar Tractor Company. Indust. Med. 15:179 (March) 1946.

Index